ADVANCES IN TESTOSTERONE ACTION

Edited by **Manuel Estrada**

Advances in Testosterone Action
http://dx.doi.org/10.5772/intechopen.72493
Edited by Manuel Estrada

Contributors

Ken-Ichi Takayama, Marcelo George Mungai Chacur, Alex Arikawa, Camila Souza, Eunice Oba, Luis Roberto Gabriel Filho, Alexander Shpakov, Julian Ryzhov, Andrey Bakhtyukov, Kira Derkach, José Macedo, Maristela Oliveira, Olga Sampaio, Maria P De Miguel, Manuel Nistal, Pilar Gonzalez-Peramato

First published in London, United Kingdom, 2018 by IntechOpen
IntechOpen is the global imprint of INTECHOPEN LIMITED, registered in England and Wales, registration number: 11086078, The Shard, 25th floor, 32 London Bridge Street
London, SE19SG – United Kingdom
Printed in Croatia

British Library Cataloguing-in-Publication Data
A catalogue record for this book is available from the British Library

Additional hard copies can be obtained from orders@intechopen.com

Advances in Testosterone Action, Edited by Manuel Estrada
p. cm.
Print ISBN 978-1-78984-512-9
Online ISBN 978-1-78984-513-6

For EU product safety concerns:
IN TECH d.o.o., Prolaz Marije Krucifikse Kozulić 3, 51000 Rijeka, Croatia,
info@intechopen.com or visit our website at intechopen.com.

Meet the editor

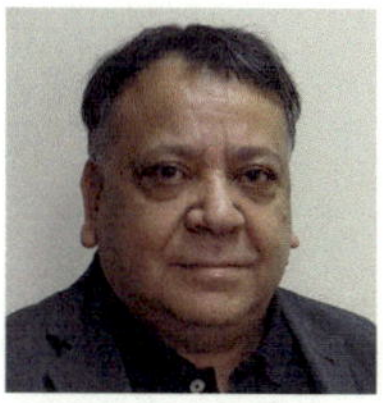

Manuel Estrada received his PhD degree in Biomedical Sciences from Universidad de Chile in 2003. From 2003 to 2006, he served as a postdoctoral fellow at the Department of Pharmacology, Medical School, at Yale University. Since 2006 he has been Associate Professor of Physiology at the Department of Physiology and Biophysics, Faculty of Medicine, Universidad de Chile. His research interests include rapid androgen effects and cardiomyocyte metabolic adaptations to hypertrophy. He is an author of many papers published in international peer-reviewed journals, and his presence is often requested as an invited speaker at congresses and diverse scientific meetings.

Contents

Preface

This book includes recent findings on androgen actions and the endocrinology field. The chapters include information in physiological and pathological conditions such as alterations in testosterone production by Leydig cells, prostate cancer, and metabolic disorders. Moreover, the book includes information regarding the potential use of androgens in assisted human reproduction treatments and bovine breeding. Each chapter contains background information based on evidence, which emphasizes basic science, aimed at professionals who already have a basic understanding of the principles of androgen biochemistry and endocrine-related diseases.

Androgens direct the differentiation of organs and tissues towards the adoption of male phenotypes. Testosterone, the main physiological male-related sex hormone, is well known for its androgenic properties and anabolic effects. Cell-specific and concentration-dependent effects are modulated through circulating plasma levels of testosterone, cell metabolism, and expression of androgen receptors. Given the important roles of androgens in normal physiology in men, abnormal levels must be considered as one of the main causes implicated in several disorders and pathological conditions.

Testosterone production is regulated through the hypothalamic–pituitary–gonad axis. The hypothalamus produces and secretes gonadotrophin-releasing hormone, which stimulates the pituitary to secrete luteinizing hormone, which then prompts the Leydig cells in the testes to produce testosterone. A reduced number of Leydig cells as well as decreased ability to respond to intracellular signaling are important factors that contribute to induce testosterone deficit in men. The chapter by De Miguel *et al.* describes and discusses the histological changes produced in human Leydig cells in both physiological and pathological conditions occurring at various times throughout life.

Metabolic disorders have been correlated with low testosterone plasma levels. Clinical trials have demonstrated that exogenous administration of testosterone at physiological concentrations improves insulin sensitivity, central obesity, and heart failure progression in men suffering from metabolic syndrome. The chapter by Shpakov *et al.* comprehensively describes new aspects of the metabolic effects of androgens and their relationship with endocrine and paracrine factors, specifically with adipokines. Adipokines are mainly produced in the liver, although several cells also express the gene for these proteins. Thus, an interesting concept is that production and secretion of adipokines could control systemic and local testosterone levels by the hypothalamic–pituitary–gonad axis.

Testosterone exerts its effects mainly by activating the androgen receptor and thereby promoting the expression of genes containing specific androgen-response elements in their promoter regions. Testosterone-regulated transcription is mediated either directly by the activated androgen receptor or by association with additional transcription factors and coregulator proteins. Prostate cancer, for example, is associated with alterations in androgen receptor functions. The chapter by Ken-ichi Takayama exhaustively reviews the current knowledge on molecular biology and pharmacology of the androgen receptor in prostate cancer. The author analyzes the new molecular actions associated with the action mechanism of androgens and the role of non-coding RNAs, such as lncRNAs and miRNAs, in prostate cancer progression.

Furthermore, this book covers the potential use of androgens in both human and bovine reproduction protocols. The chapter by De Macedo *et al.* describes the effect of dehydroepiandrosterone supplementation as an adjunct in ovarian stimulation procedures used in assisted human reproduction treatments. Recent research has indicated that treatment of patients with low antral follicle counts with moderate doses of androgens can increase both the quantity and quality of oocytes and embryos, leading to favorable results in assisted human reproduction treatments. Finally, the chapter by Chacur *et al.* shows correlations between circulating testosterone concentrations and reproductive tract morphometry variables, which are useful in practical settings and in the selection of young bulls bred in extensive management feeding, therefore providing new knowledge in the field of bovine reproduction.

These recent findings motivated us to explore whether appropriate testosterone signaling through new endocrine players might explain both physiological and adverse roles of androgens. I hope that this book will provide the reader with a current overview of the actions and potential use of androgens.

Manuel Estrada
Programa de Fisiología y Biofísica
Facultad de Medicina
Universidad de Chile
Santiago, Chile

Chapter 1

Morphological Bases of Human Leydig Cell Dysfunction

Maria P. De Miguel, Pilar Gonzalez-Peramato and
Manuel Nistal

Additional information is available at the end of the chapter

http://dx.doi.org/10.5772/intechopen.79201

Abstract

In this chapter, we describe the histophysiology of human Leydig cells, their cytological characteristics, their differentiation processes, and the physiopathological processes occurring at various times throughout life. We first focus on the normal development of fetal Leydig cells as well as the pathologies of fetal Leydig cells that can affect numbers or hyperplasic processes (e.g., hypogonadotropic hypogonadism, cryptorchidism, congenital Leydig cell hyperplasia secondary to diabetes, and isoimmunization). Next, we explain the changes occurring at puberty with the onset and differentiation of adult Leydig cells and the pathophysiology of delayed puberty. We then describe the histophysiology of adult Leydig cells and the most frequent pathologies (e.g., hypogonadotropic hypogonadism, testicular dysgenesia, mild androgen insensitivity syndrome, 5-α-reductase defect, and Klinefelter syndrome). Finally, we discuss the morphological changes of these cells in the elderly.

Keywords: fetal Leydig cells, adult Leydig cells, testosterone, puberty, elderly, dysgenesia, pathology

1. Introduction

Leydig cells are the primary producers of testosterone. They perform important functions during fetal life, in the first months of life, and in adults, ranging from male sexual differentiation and testicular descent to the acquisition of a normal number of spermatogonial stem cells, the development of spermatogenesis and thus fertility, and the maintenance of typical male characteristics in adulthood.

2. Fetal stage

2.1. Origin and development of fetal Leydig cells

During development, two different types of Leydig cells appear sequentially, fetal Leydig cells and adult Leydig cells, which display different functional characteristics, reflecting their morphology, steroid capacity, and regulatory mechanisms. Fetal Leydig cells are detected immediately after gonadal sex differentiation [1]. Adult Leydig cells begin to develop at the beginning of puberty and acquire their maximum numbers at the end of puberty. The origin of both Leydig cell types is debated: some suggest a parent-common progenitor pool in the fetal testis [2, 3] and others have suggested that Leydig cells in adults might originate in precursors to fetal Leydig cells [4]. In addition, a three-phase model of the development of Leydig cells has been proposed: fetal, neonatal, and adult Leydig cells [5].

2.1.1. Development of fetal Leydig cells

The mesonephros and the coelomic epithelium are considered the two most plausible origins of fetal Leydig cells. The progenitor cells expressing SF1 actively proliferate and ultimately lose this marker when cell differentiation begins in week 8 of human gestation. The first sign of differentiation is the histochemical detection of 3-beta hydroxysteroid dehydrogenase (3β-HSD) in the cytoplasm. About 83% of 3β-HSD-positive cells show a high intensity of androgen receptors (ARs) immunoreaction.

Fetal Leydig cells express various steroidogenic enzymes required for androgen synthesis, such as acute regulatory protein, CYP11A1 (P450 side chain cleavage), CYP17A1 (P450C17), and 3β-HSD. The most important androgenic product of fetal Leydig cells is androstenedione. Fetal Sertoli cells make testosterone from androstenedione through the enzyme 17-β hydroxysteroid dehydrogenase (HSD17β3) at this stage of fetal testis development. Differentiation of fetal Leydig cells has been a subject of debate in recent decades and appears to be an androgen-independent process [6]. Their proliferation and subsequent development do so under the stimulus of human chorionic gonadotropin (hCG) in the first half of the gestation period and with the help of luteinizing hormone (LH) secreted by the pituitary gland in the last half. Both hormones are glycoproteic in nature and act through the same receptor (LHCGR).

2.1.2. Evolution throughout fetal life

Fetal Leydig cells are identified by positivity for the 3β-HSD enzyme. The maximum peak of Leydig cell numbers is reached at week 19 of gestation (**Figure 1**). Remarkably, this peak occurs in parallel with the disappearance of one of the two layers of peritubular cells of the seminiferous epithelium, the outermost layer of peritubular cells, between weeks 17 and 19 of gestation. These two occurrences also match the maximum production of testosterone between the 14th and 19th weeks of fetal life. After a few weeks of Leydig cell quiescence, from week 22 of gestation, a progressive decrease in the number of Leydig cells is observed.

Most fetal Leydig cells disappear after birth; however, a subpopulation persists in the postnatal testis that is estimated to represent 10% of all Leydig cells in adulthood [7–9]. Given that

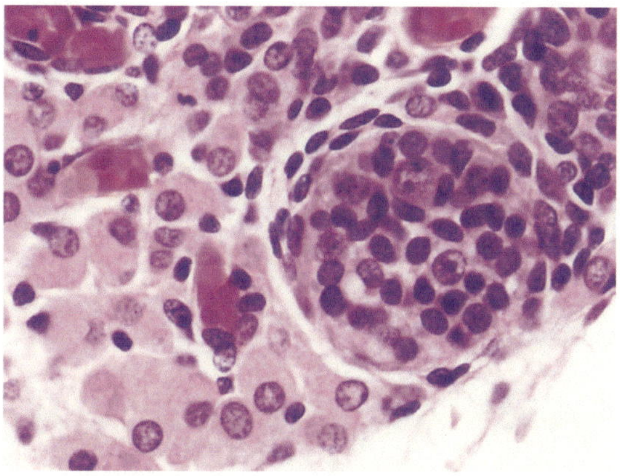

Figure 1. Fetus at 19 weeks. Seminiferous tube showing two gonocytes in the center, with the remaining cells, the Sertoli cells. In the interstitium, Leydig cells with peripheral nuclei and broad eosinophilic cytoplasm are abundantly found.

fetal Leydig cells do not express HSD17β3, they cannot directly synthesize testosterone; thus, their functional importance in adults is unknown.

2.2. Functions of fetal Leydig cells

2.2.1. *Differentiation of the genitals*

Under the action of testosterone, the differentiation of the Wolff tubes takes place. This differentiation is ipsilateral and gives rise to the development of the epididymis, vas deferens, and seminal vesicle. When testosterone is converted into dihydrotestosterone by the enzyme 5-α-reductase, differentiation of the prostate and development of the external genitalia occur: male urethra, penis, and scrotum.

2.2.2. *Testicular descent*

The two stages of testicular descent, transabdominal and inguinoscrotal, are controlled directly or indirectly by fetal Leydig cells. Transabdominal descent depends on an androgen-independent peptide, insulin-like growth factor 3 (INLS3), whereas inguinoscrotal descent is mediated by androgens through the masculinization they produce in the genitofemoral nerve neurons. Those neurons produce calcitonin gene-related peptide (CGRP), which is responsible for the development that the gubernaculum acquires, allowing testicle descent [10].

2.3. Pathology of fetal Leydig cells

2.3.1. *Defective androgen synthesis*

Defects in the synthesis of androgens due to various autosomal hereditary syndromes result in absent or incomplete virilization. They include lipoid congenital adrenal hyperplasia (lipoid CAH), deficits in 3-βHSD/17,20-lyase, α-hydroxylase 17/17,20-lyase deficiency, deficit in 17,20 desmolase, and deficit in 17-β hydroxysteroid dehydrogenase.

2.3.1.1. *Lipoid CAH*

It is the most severe form of congenital adrenal hyperplasia. It affects the synthesis of adrenal and gonadal steroid hormones. Genetically 46,XY patients are phenotypically women with severe salt-losing syndrome. There is no uniformity in the histological descriptions of the Leydig cells; in some cases, they are described as having large accumulations of lipids [11], whereas in others, such lipid inclusions are absent [12].

2.3.1.2. *3-βHSD/17,20-lyase deficit*

Patients with a mild deficiency have normal external genitalia; some consult for hypospadias or micropenis [13], and the testicles are smaller than normal.

2.3.1.3. *17-α Hydroxylase/17,20-lyase deficiency*

Patients have a significant degree of undermasculinization; they can even mature as girls and consult at puberty for amenorrhea. The testes show a delay in pubertal development and hyperplasia of Leydig cells.

2.3.1.4. *17,20 Desmolase deficit*

It presents with a high variability in external genital development, from a female phenotype to males with micropenis that is hardly virilized, bifid scrotum, perineal hypospadias, and cryptorchidism, due to the insufficient production of testosterone during fetal life.

2.3.1.5. *17-β-Hydroxysteroid dehydrogenase deficit*

Patients show a female phenotype at birth, grow up as girls, and suffer significant virilization at puberty. The cryptorchid testis or testis housed in the labia majora has low spermatogenesis development, testicular mixed atrophy, Sertoli cell-only testis histology, and in all cases, Leydig cell hyperplasia [14].

2.3.2. *Hypoplasia of Leydig cells*

Inactivating mutations in the LHCGR gene, primarily those involving amino acid sequences, result in a rare 46,XY disorder in sexual development (DSD) [15]. A spectrum of phenotypes can occur, ranging from a severe form with a female phenotype (Leydig cell hypoplasia (LCH) type I) when various mutations, deletions, or insertions produce a complete inactivation of LHCGR to a milder form of LCH (type II) when some receptor activity is maintained with male undervirilization (delayed puberty, primary hypogonadism, micropenis, or hypospadias) [16]. The testes in patients with LCH type I remain in the adult as a pattern of infant development with an absence of germ cells and Leydig cells. The epididymides and vas deferens are absent or hypoplastic. In patients with LCH type II, a pattern similar to the previous one has been reported, with the presence of small groups of Leydig cells and focal spermatogenesis [17].

2.3.3. *Transient androgenic insufficiency*

Testicular descent is a complex process in which multiple factors are involved sequentially and synergistically, highlighting the role of the hypothalamic-pituitary-testicular axis. Congenital cryptorchidism has been linked to a hormonal dysfunction, emphasizing the role of testosterone. Androgenic insufficiency during the second and third trimesters of pregnancy secondary to poor stimulation of the Leydig cells either by the pituitary hormones or by HCG has been suggested. This insufficiency might be low and transient given that no other genital anomalies except epididymal anomalies are present [18].

2.3.4. *Congenital hyperplasia of Leydig cells*

The presence in the newborn of a nodular or a diffuse Leydig hyperplasia is most often due to hyperstimulation by the mother's hCG, which, under certain conditions, can pass to the fetus in large quantities (**Figure 2**).

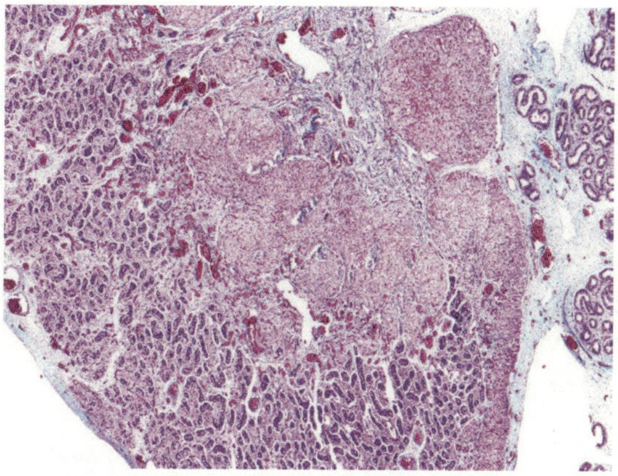

Figure 2. Congenital Leydig cell hyperplasia in a son of a mother with diabetes. Several nodules of Leydig cells are observed located in the testicular mediastinum and subalbuginea region.

Children of mothers with diabetes who have very edematous placentas could suffer this phenomenon. It has also been observed in triploid fetuses, in newborns with Beckwitz-Wiedemann syndrome, nonimmune hydrops fetalis, Rh isoimmunization or leprechaunism, and in complicated pregnancies [19].

3. Neonatal stage

3.1. Mini-puberty

In the first few months of postnatal life, a second wave of Leydig cell proliferation occurs (**Figure 3**), which depends on a transient reactivation of the hypothalamic-pituitary-testicular axis that begins immediately after birth. This stage is known as mini-puberty and begins with

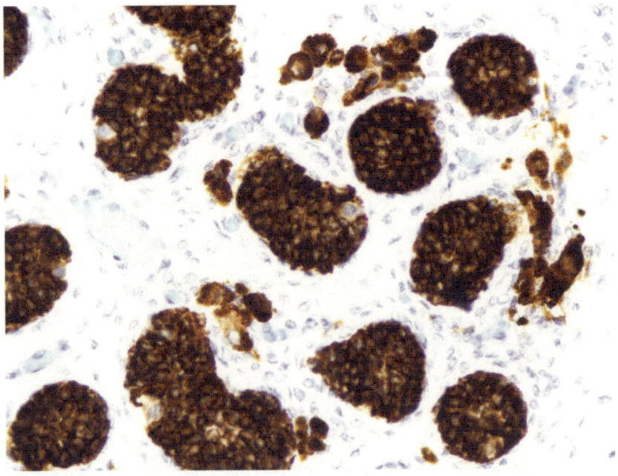

Figure 3. Infant of 3.5 months of age. The testicular parenchyma shows small clusters of Leydig cells between the seminiferous tubules. Immunostaining for inhibin in brown.

an elevation in LH and follicle-stimulating hormone (FSH). Then, an increase in the number of Leydig cells reaches a peak in the third month after birth, and secondarily, an increase in the production of testosterone and estradiol [20]. This transient stimulation determines important changes in the various cells of the testicle. An increase in the number of Sertoli cells ensuring normal spermatogenesis in adult life [21] and a transformation of gonocytes into adult spermatogonia reaches a peak by postnatal day 100. Six months after birth, coinciding with the decrease in GnRH pulses, a loss of germ cells then begins. Outside the genital tract, mini-puberty is key to the masculinization of the brain.

3.2. Pathology of mini-puberty

The most frequent pathology at this stage of development is hypogonadotropic hypogonadism, which is transient in most patients with undescended testes and permanent in other conditions such as Kallmann syndrome, multiple pituitary hormone deficiency, and DAX-1 mutations [22]. The lack of gonocyte differentiation into adult spermatogonia can be the cause of many infertility disorders that have been considered idiopathic until now.

4. Childhood

After mini-puberty, the testicle enters a resting phase that lasts until the end of the third year of life. During this period, most fetal Leydig cells involute and disappear [8]. At the beginning of the fourth year, coinciding with the activation of the androgenic receptors in the Sertoli cells, a wave of proliferation and differentiation of the germ cells begins in the seminiferous tubules. This wave is observed at the appearance of various types of spermatogonia and type I spermatocytes. The purpose of this process is not well understood, but it leads to a renewal of the germ cells. After a short time, the most differentiated cells (the spermatocytes) undergo apoptosis and are phagocytosed by Sertoli cells. Until the beginning of puberty, no Leydig cells are observed in the interstitium but are represented by fibroblastic-like cells with some lipid vacuoles.

The most frequent pathology of Leydig cells during this period is a persistence of abundant fetal Leydig cells and Leydig cell hyperplasia.

4.1. Persistence of fetal Leydig cells

The persistence of isolated fetal Leydig cells throughout childhood and even in adult testes is a normal occurrence. In any case, it is an androgen-independent subpopulation [9]. What is pathological is the presence of abundant Leydig cell clusters that also show a large cytoplasmic vacuolization due to the presence of abundant lipid inclusions. Most patients with these alterations are DSD carriers. The persistence of fetal Leydig cells is characteristic of the testis of patients with DSD with NR5A1 gene mutations (**Figure 4**), congenital lipoid adrenal hyperplasia (due to StAR mutations) [23], or a deficit of 5α-reductase and androgen insensitivity. These alterations are remarkable in the first years of life.

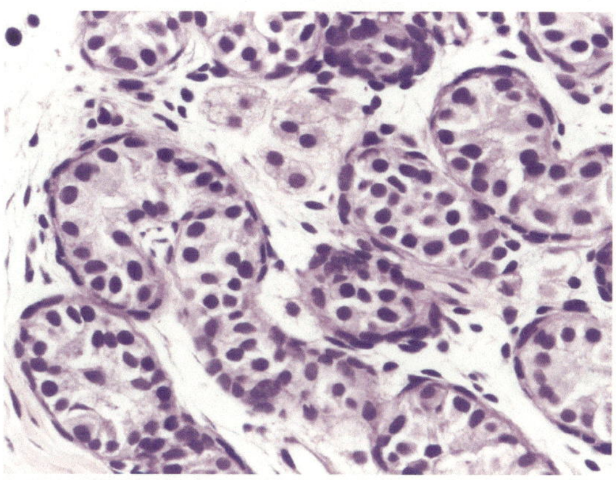

Figure 4. Patient with 46,XY DSD by mutation in the NR5A1 gene, showing Leydig cells in clusters and isolated between seminiferous tubules with a few germ cells showing highly vacuolated cytoplasms due to the high lipid content.

4.2. Hyperplasia of Leydig cells

The presence of abundant Leydig cells in childhood is a rare occurrence and is clinically manifested by symptoms of precocious puberty. It is observed in familial testotoxicosis, in some cases of McCune-Albright syndrome (MAS), Leydig cell hyperplasia/Leydig cell tumor, and extratesticular hCG-secreting tumors.

4.2.1. Familial testotoxicosis

It is also known as gonadotropin-independent precocious puberty (GIPP) or familial male-limited precocious puberty (FMPP) and is an autosomal-dominant disorder caused by a constitutive activating mutation of the LH/CGR gene [24]. It is a form of precocious male puberty characterized by the early maturation of Leydig cells and spermatogenesis in the absence of pituitary gonadotropic stimulation [25] (**Figure 5**).

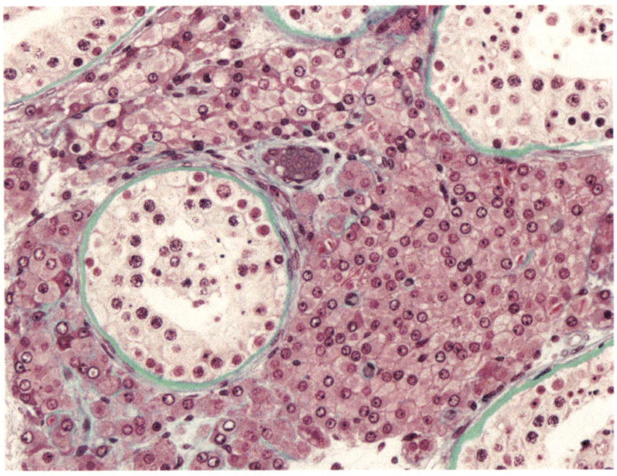

Figure 5. Hyperplasia of Leydig cells surrounded by seminiferous tubules with spermatogenesis in a 3-year-old patient with testotoxicosis.

4.2.2. McCune-Albright syndrome

It is considered an example of mixed peripheral and early precocious puberty. This syndrome is characterized by polyostotic fibrous dysplasia, "*café au lait*" skin pigmentation, and autonomous endocrine hyperfunction. At the testicular level, it is manifested by a secondary macroorchidism, in some cases associated with isolated hyperfunction of the Sertoli cells, and in other cases to a hyperfunction of the Leydig cells without the activation of the Sertoli cells [26].

4.2.3. Leydig cell hyperplasia/Leydig cell tumor

More frequently than the above situations, hyperplasia of Leydig cells in childhood is observed, which manifests clinically with the same symptoms as functioning Leydig cell tumors. Histologically, there are several nodules of hypertrophic Leydig cells located between or surrounded by seminiferous tubules with complete spermatogenesis. Whether Leydig cell hyperplasia with focal spermatogenesis in childhood is a precursor lesion of some tumors of Leydig cells is a matter of debate.

4.2.4. Leydig cell hyperplasia secondary to extratesticular hCG-secreting tumors

Numerous extratesticular tumors have been described (mediastinal, retroperitoneal, basal ganglia, pineal, or suprasellar region) that manifest with precocious pseudopuberty. All are hCG secretors. Leydig cell hyperplasia is mostly moderate but could be responsible for complete spermatogenesis [27].

5. Puberty

5.1. Differentiation of adult Leydig cells

The onset of puberty depends on both genetic and environmental factors. Under the action of gonadotropin-releasing hypothalamic hormone (GnRH), gonadotropic cell receptors of the anterior lobe of the pituitary gland are stimulated, and the synthesis of FSH and LH begins. The onset of puberty occurs around the age of 9 years. Adult Leydig cells originate at the onset of puberty after an active proliferation of undifferentiated stem cells. Under the stimulus of LH, these cells first become stellate or spindle-shaped, from either the tubular or perivascular wall, and begin to show steroidogenic activity. Initially, as immature cells, they produce 5-α-reduced androgens more than testosterone, and later when they have acquired a polyhedral shape, the mature cells produce testosterone. Leydig cells are arranged isolated or in small groups between the seminiferous tubules, which in turn are increasingly developing the germ line, in a proportion estimated at 1.2 groups (regardless of the number of cells) per cross-tubular section. The change in testicular size is rapid and detectable at an average age of 13.5 years and is followed 1 or 2 years later by an increase in body height and the development of male secondary sexual characteristics.

5.2. Delay in the differentiation of adult Leydig cells

The most frequent pathology observed during puberty is a delay in the differentiation of Leydig cells. This delay causes an absence of or low testosterone levels, and as a consequence, a serious defect in spermatogenesis in the testicle occurs that is clinically expressed as delayed puberty. Delayed puberty is suspected when at the age of 14 years, the testis has not reached 3 ml of volume and its major axis is less than 2.5 cm. If the defect persists beyond 18 years, the patient probably carries a form of hypogonadotropic hypogonadism.

5.2.1. Constitutional delay of growth and puberty (CDGP)

Delayed puberty is a symptom for which adolescents are frequently sent to the endocrinologist, considered a minor GnRH deficit [28]. Many cases are inherited as an autosomal-dominant, -recessive, or X-linked trait. It is twice as frequent in boys as in girls. Although delayed puberty has multiple possible causes, the conjunction of elevated serum ghrelin and low concentrations of leptin is worth noting. Histologically, the testes remain prepubertal; no tubular development and adult Leydig cells are observed.

5.2.2. Delayed puberty associated with chronic illness

A number of situations can lead to delayed puberty, from malnutrition to chronic diseases (e.g., gastrointestinal diseases, chronic anemia, recurrent infections, immunodeficiency, respiratory diseases, and endocrine diseases). Even excessive exercise at this age could be a cause. The testis in most cases shows isolated small-sized Leydig cells with poor immunostaining for testosterone.

6. Adulthood

6.1. Histophysiology of adult Leydig cells

Leydig cells represent 3.8% of the testicular volume [29]. As polyhedral cells arranged in isolation or in small clusters (**Figure 6**), they are frequently observed in the tunica propria of the

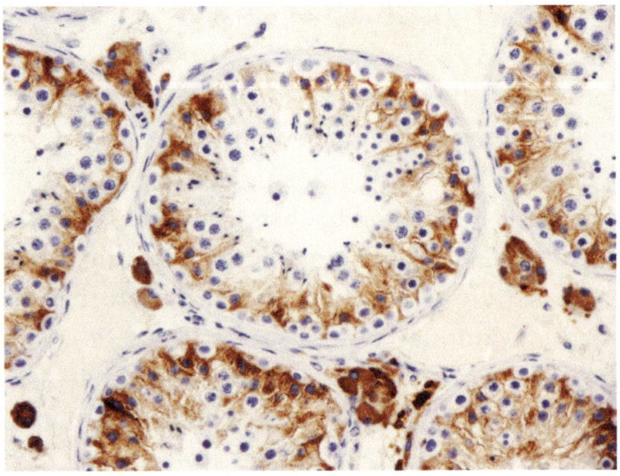

Figure 6. Transverse sections of seminiferous tubules with complete spermatogenesis in an adult patient. Immunostaining for inhibin highlights both Sertoli cell and Leydig cell clusters in the interstitium.

seminiferous tubules (peritubular Leydig cells) and as ectopic cells (testicular mediastinum, interlobular septa, albuginea, epididymis, and spermatic cord).

Cellular characteristics include an eosinophilic cytoplasm and an eccentric nucleus with one or two nucleoli. In the cytoplasm, the machinery is at the service of the transformation of cholesterol into testosterone, which includes the presence of abundant lipid droplets, significant development of the smooth endoplasmic reticulum, mitochondria with tubular crests, peroxisomes, and lipofuscins. Many cells contain Reinke crystals as well. Leydig cell clusters are joined by gap junctions.

The proper function of Leydig cells depends not only on the presence of LH receptors but a complex paracrine network in which Sertoli cells, germ cells, peritubular cells, macrophages, telocytes, and even vascular endothelial cells are involved [30]. Leydig cells show morphological changes in relation to the six stages of the cycle of the human seminiferous epithelium [29]. In adulthood, they rarely show mitosis [31]. Their numbers begin to decrease slowly after puberty, and at 60 years, there are approximately half as many as at age 20. However, the production of testosterone is maintained well until the end of the fifth decade due to the high number of cells.

6.2. Pathology of adult Leydig cells

6.2.1. Alterations in number

6.2.1.1. Absence or incomplete maturation of Leydig cells

It is the characteristic histological picture of most hypogonadotropic hypogonadisms (HHs). They include normosmic idiopathic HH, HH with anosmia or Kallmann syndrome, and HH due to LH deficiency. Another situation in which a small number of Leydig cells are observed occurs when LH is biologically inactive.

The most frequent genetic anomalies identified as causes of normosmic idiopathic HH are those in genes related to the synthesis and secretion of GnRH, such as GNRHR/GNRH1, TAC3/TACR3, KISS1R and KISS1, FGFR1 and CHD7. In the HH associated with anosmia described by [32] and many years later known as Kallmann syndrome, KAL1 gene mutations are predominant. In these two types of hypogonadism, serum determinations of FSH and LH are very low or undetectable. The testicles show a childhood or a pubertal development pattern depending on the complete or partial absence of GnRH. In the first case, a testicular interstitium in which Leydig cells and their precursors are absent or are undetectable (**Figure 7**) is worth noting. In the second case, in which patients have a low GnRH, they present pulsatile secretions of FSH and LH that ensure maturation of isolated Leydig cells and then some secretion of testosterone allowing for testicular development that is closer to that of a pubertal testis [33, 34].

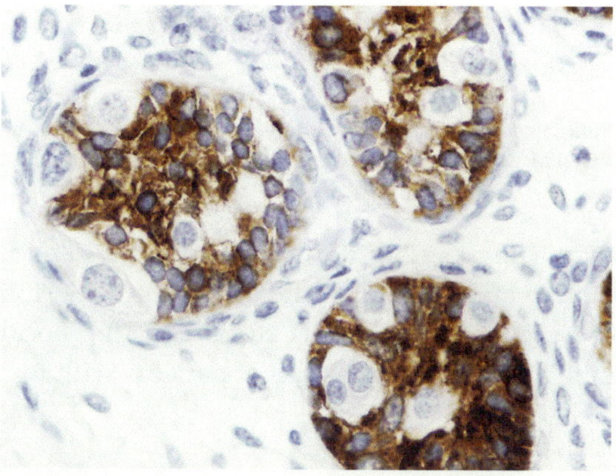

Figure 7. Adult patient of 26 years with hypogonadotropic hypogonadism with anosmia (Kallmann's syndrome). The interstitium shows a complete absence of Leydig cells. At the tubular level, binucleated spermatogonia and intense immunostaining for inhibin are observed in the cytoplasm of Sertoli cells.

In the isolated LH deficit (Pasqualini-Bur-McCullagh syndrome, fertile eunuch syndrome), serum levels of FSH are normal, whereas those of LH and testosterone are very low [35]. In some cases, the cause is a mutation in both the LH β subunit gene and in the gonadotropin-releasing hormone receptor. The testicles present complete but quantitatively abnormal spermatogenesis at the tubular level with a depopulated interstitium or very few Leydig cells. A minimum production of testosterone and a proper functioning of Sertoli cells needed for spermatogenesis are achieved. Among the many complex syndromes in which this deficit in the development of Leydig cells can be seen are Prader-Willi syndrome, Bardet-Biedl syndrome, Biemond syndrome, Frasser syndrome, and hypogonadism associated with dermatological diseases, ataxia, or central demyelination.

6.2.1.2. Focal hyperplasia of Leydig cells

It is a very common condition in ex-cryptorchid testicles, in infertile patients, and in peritumoral parenchyma that has been conserved in germ cell tumors. The focal hyperplasia is defined by the presence of clusters of at least 14 Leydig cells and by the fact that they do not distort the testicular architecture, conserving the seminiferous tubules without englobing them. Focal hyperplasia is typically associated with poor spermatogenesis (**Figure 8**). Patients frequently suffer a decrease in testosterone/LH ratio and testosterone/estradiol ratio. The presence of a focal hyperplasia of the Leydig cells represents a loss of the normal paracrine

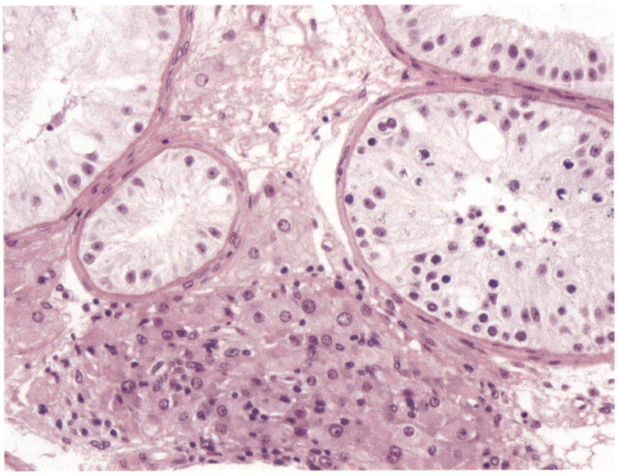

Figure 8. Focal nodular hyperplasia of Leydig cells in an adult male aged 30 years with cryptorchidism. Testicular parenchyma with mixed atrophy shows tubules with spermatogenesis and tubules with only Sertoli cells.

interactions between Sertoli cells, peritubular myoid cells, and Leydig cells. Some believe it to be the result of a defect in fetal life that probably depends on Sertoli cells, given that Sertoli cells are responsible for the quantity of Leydig stem cells [36]. Focal hyperplasia of Leydig cells is included among the most frequent lesions of patients with testicular dysgenesis [37].

6.2.1.3. *Diffuse hyperplasia of Leydig cells*

With this condition, Leydig cells are not only increased in number (hyperplasia) but often show hypertrophy. This hyperplasia is observed in patients with androgen insensitivity, a defect in 5-α reductase, DSD with dysgenetic testis, in many infertile patients of uncertain etiology and between the conserved seminiferous tubules of a testicle carrying a germ-cell tumor secreting β-hCG or even in the contralateral testis of such tumor.

The androgen resistance syndromes are a group of DSDs characterized by a 46,XY karyotype and phenotypes ranging from female (testicular feminization) to normal males who consult for infertility. The cause must be found in one of the almost 1000 mutations described in the AR gene. The three main forms, CAIS (complete testicular feminization), PAIS (partial testicular feminization), and MAIS (slight or minimal androgen insensitivity) [38], have been described according to the phenotype. The complete form is rarely diagnosed in childhood; patients consult for amenorrhea, or the testicles are an incidental finding during a herniorrhaphy. PAIS is diagnosed more often in childhood, associated with surgical interventions for the reconstruction of the external genitalia. Patients with CAIS and PAIS have a pathognomonic histological image: a testicular interstitium populated by numerous Leydig cells next to the seminiferous tubules, which, due to the absence of androgenic receptors in Sertoli cells, remain at infantile development (**Figure 9**). The Leydig cells usually do not show hyperplasia; many have hyperchromatic nuclei and/or abundant cytoplasmic vacuoles. Two-thirds of the testicles have Sertoli/Leydig hamartomas, which are nonencapsulated nodular formations constituted by parenchyma similar to the rest of the testicle.

Patients with MAIS frequently consult for infertility. They are phenotypically males with minimal malformations of the external genitalia, simple coronal hypospadias, or a prominent midline

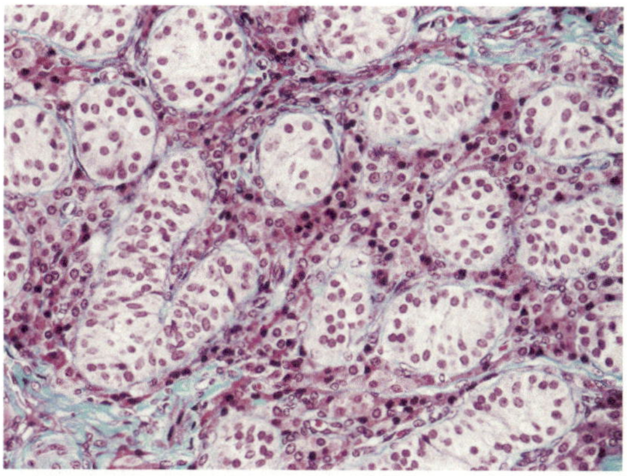

Figure 9. Patient of 20 years with 46,XY DSD with complete androgen insensitivity. The diffuse Leydig cells hyperplasia contrasts with the prepubertal development of the seminiferous tubules.

raphe of the scrotum. On the biopsy, a diffuse hyperplasia of Leydig cells surrounding each of the seminiferous tubules is observed. The presence of spermatogenesis varies from case to case [39].

Patients with a defect in 5-α reductase rarely show spermatogenesis, and the seminiferous epithelium is reduced to only Sertoli cells with incomplete maturation. The interstitium contains an elevated number of Leydig cells whose morphology is apparently normal.

In adult patients with dysgenetic testis secondary to an abnormal secretion or action of the anti-Müllerian hormone (AMH) (Sohval syndrome, male dysgenetic pseudohermaphroditism, and male with uterus), the function of Leydig cells is poor and many patients have hypergonadotropic hypogonadism. Leydig cells are not only increased in number in the interstitium but it is worth noting that a high number of Leydig cells are peritubular, forming rings in between the tubular wall (**Figure 10**).

In the testicular tumors secreting β-hCG, a marked diffuse hyperplasia of Leydig cells is generally observed. In some cases, and coinciding with burned-out tumors, Leydig cells are not only increased

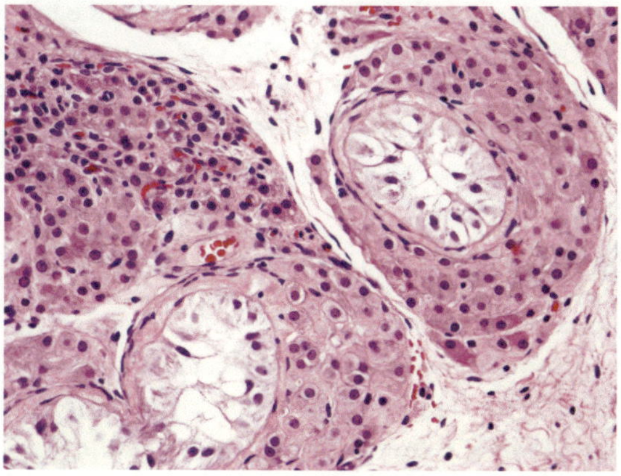

Figure 10. Male pseudohermaphroditism patient with dysgenetic testes. Note the presence of concentric rings of Leydig cells in the thickness of the tubular wall.

in number but their cytoplasm is balonized and does not show its characteristic eosinophilia. The appearance of a high number of macrophage clusters between the Leydig cells is common.

6.2.1.4. Nodular hyperplasia of Leydig cells

The presence of Leydig cell nodules has classically been considered as one of the more common histologic features in patients with 47,XXY Klinefelter syndrome. The pathology is associated with a diffuse tubular hyalinization with or without the presence of isolated tubules with only Sertoli cells or with spermatogenesis (**Figure 11**).

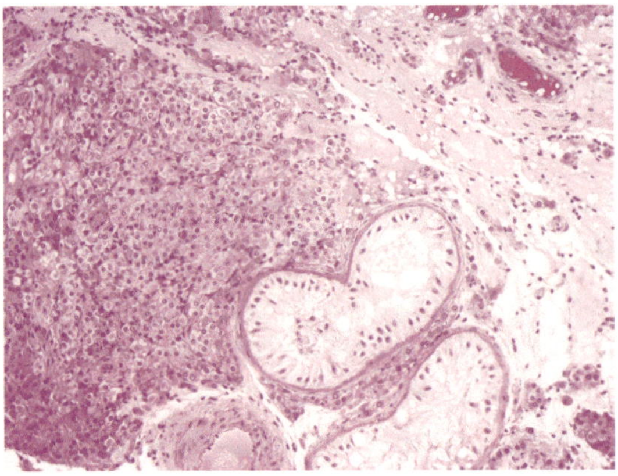

Figure 11. Klinefelter syndrome in a 32-year-old patient who consulted for infertility. Next to a nodular Leydig cells, hyperplasia seminiferous tubules with only Sertoli cells and sclerotic tubules are observed.

This form of hyperplasia is more about histological appearance than actual hyperplasia, if we consider the small size of the testicles and the disappearance of the seminiferous tubules. Both quantitative and qualitative studies have concluded that the number of Leydig cells is not increased [40]. The population of Leydig cells present is also not uniform. There are hypertrophic cells, involuted cells, and immature cells [41]. In most variants of Klinefelter syndrome, such as those with karyotypes 46,XX / 47,XYY, 48,XXYY, 48,XXXY, and 49,XXXY, Leydig cell hyperplasia is less important and can be both nodular and diffuse [42]. The 46,XX males with a normal phenotype and normal external genitalia and most patients with microdeletions of the AZF region of the Y chromosome also present Leydig cell hyperplasia that is frequently diffuse [43].

6.2.2. Alterations in Leydig cell location

There are two different situations in testicular pathology in which Leydig cells do not have a direct relationship with Sertoli cells: when they are located in the perilobular area and when they are inside the seminiferous tubules. Perilobular distribution refers to the presence of Leydig cells surrounding each testis lobule (**Figure 12**), characteristic of patients with androgen insensitivity, although it is probably a diffuse hyperplasia that isolates the seminiferous tubules.

The other location is inside seminiferous tubules, which have frequently lost the seminiferous epithelium (**Figure 13**). This ectopic location is associated with tubular dysgenesia, such as

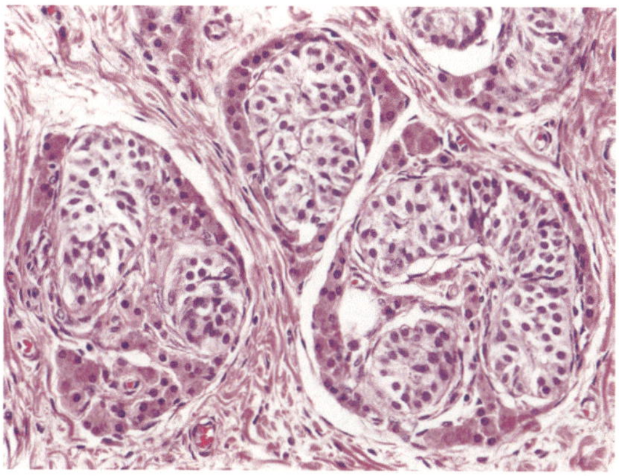

Figure 12. Preferential perilobular distribution of Leydig cells in a patient with complete androgen insensitivity. Abundant fibrosis in the interstitium stands out.

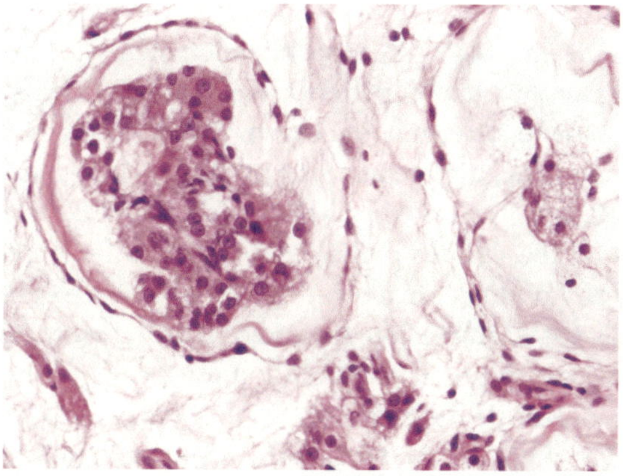

Figure 13. Leydig cells inside the sections of two seminiferous tubules in a 42-year-old patient with cryptorchidism. In contrast with atrophic characteristics of interstitial Leydig cells, normal-looking or xantomized Leydig cells in intratubular location can be observed.

Klinefelter syndrome, cryptorchid testicles that do not descend until adult age, and in some infertile patients. In many cases, the intratubular Leydig cells are accompanied by blood vessels, probably representing a migration of both Leydig cells and blood vessels normally present in the tubular wall to the interior once the cells of the seminiferous epithelium disappear.

6.2.3. *Qualitative alterations*

Among these alterations are Leydig cells with signs of hypertrophy, xantomized cytoplasm, and the presence of lamellar inclusions in the cytoplasm.

6.2.3.1. *Cellular hypertrophy*

It is common in most cases of hyperplasia; however, various degrees of cell hypertrophy with normal Leydig cell groups can coexist in the same testis. *Cytoplasmic xantomization* is always associated with cellular hypertrophy (**Figure 14**). The appearance of a pale cytoplasm with multiple

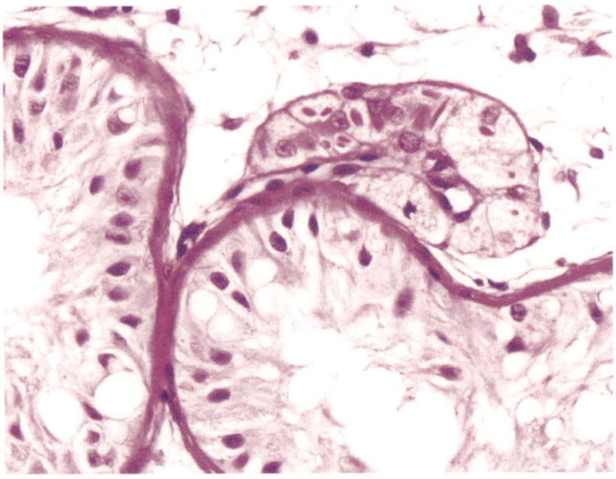

Figure 14. Testicular biopsy of an azoospermic patient. A cluster of Leydig cells with markedly xantomized cytoplasm with persistence of some Reinke crystals is shown. The nuclei of some cells are pyknotic and retracted. The neighboring seminiferous tubules lack a germ line.

small vacuoles expresses the unusually high accumulation of lipids. The cells are arranged singly or in clusters and are frequently found in patients with cryptorchidism, in DSD with dysgenetic testes, in some infertile patients, and in some elderly patients. The fact that these Leydig cells very often present with retracted, hyperchromatic nuclei in which it is difficult to recognize the nucleolus suggests that these cells have completed their biological cycle and degenerates in this way. The relationship with the various pathologies in which they are more frequently found makes it possible that many of them are dysgenetic. The presence of lamellar inclusions in the cytoplasm of Leydig cells is a characteristic feature of patients with adrenoleukodystrophy. In the variety of adrenoleukodystrophy termed adrenomyeloneuropathy, symptoms of gonadal dysfunction (loss of libido, erectile dysfunction, scant pubic hair, gynecomastia, and testicular atrophy) are observed. The patients also show a decreased seminal volume, oligozoospermia, and elevated FSH and LH. In the testis, there is severe and progressive damage of the seminiferous epithelium and alterations in Leydig cells, such as the appearance of lamellar cytoplasmic inclusions similar to the ones in adrenal cortex cells and cerebral cells [44].

7. Elderly patients

7.1. Late-onset hypogonadism

Age negatively affects all functions of the male genital tract, especially after age 65, with large inter-individual differences. Various terms have been proposed to describe this situation as "andropause," "male climacteric," "aging male syndrome," or "symptomatic" androgen deficiency in aging men. "Late-onset hypogonadism" (LOH) has been considered the most appropriate term [45, 46]. LOH is a clinical and biochemical syndrome secondary to a decrease in the serum levels of free testosterone (total testosterone will still be preserved in serum two or three decades longer). This late hypogonadism is already present in 3.1–7.0% of men between 30 and 69 years of age, but it is found in 18.4% of those over 70 years. The minimum criteria for diagnosis have been established when three clinical symptoms are present: decreased libido, morning erection, and erectile dysfunction associated with a total testosterone level of less than 11 nml/L and a free testosterone level of less than 220 pmol/L [47, 48]. Hypogonadism in some cases has been described as primary and in others as secondary.

7.2. Interpretation of elder testis histology

Assessment of Leydig cells in the elderly is complicated, and it is often difficult to distinguish between what might be considered a consequence of normal aging of the Leydig cells and what is pathological. Sometimes, the cause is local (varicocele, obstruction of the spermatic tract), and other times, it is systemic (the impact of ischemia in a complicated arteriosclerosis, hypertension or in chronic diseases and their treatments).

7.2.1. Primary alterations

Primary alterations of Leydig cells consubstantial with physiological aging are as follows: a decrease in number, the tendency to form small clusters, cellular atrophy, abundant intranuclear inclusions, multinucleation [49] (**Figure 15**), an increase in lipofuscins, an increase in lipids, immunoexpression of keratins (**Figure 16**), and a decreased immunohistochemical expression of testosterone. The number of Leydig cells at the age of 70 is less than half than at 20 years. The tendency to form clusters becomes more important in the peripheral zones of the parenchyma, under the albuginea and in the proximities of the testicular mediastinum. The cellular atrophy is revealed by pyknotic nuclei, irregular nuclear contours, and reductions in the size of the cytoplasm [50, 51]. Multinucleation appears around the age of 60 but is isolated; it is very frequent toward the age of 70, and from this age, multinucleated cells can be observed in more than half of the microscopic fields at high magnification [52]. Not all multinucleated cells are Leydig cells; an important percentage of them are telocytes (CD34-positive fibroblasts). Paracrystalline inclusions become more abundant and are frequently observed inside the nucleus [53]. The increase in lipofuscins is progressive and appears in both single-nucleated and multinucleated cells [54]. The increase in lipid vacuoles and the scarce immunostaining for testosterone is related to involutive changes in the structures

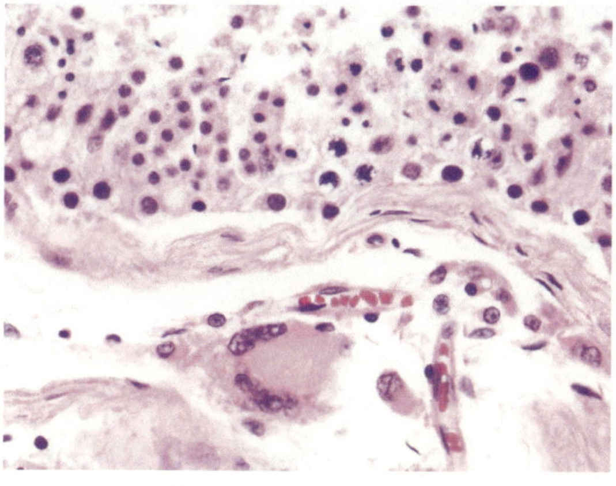

Figure 15. Multinucleated Leydig cell with typical horseshoe nuclei. Autopsy finding of a 65-year-old patient who died of myocardial infarction.

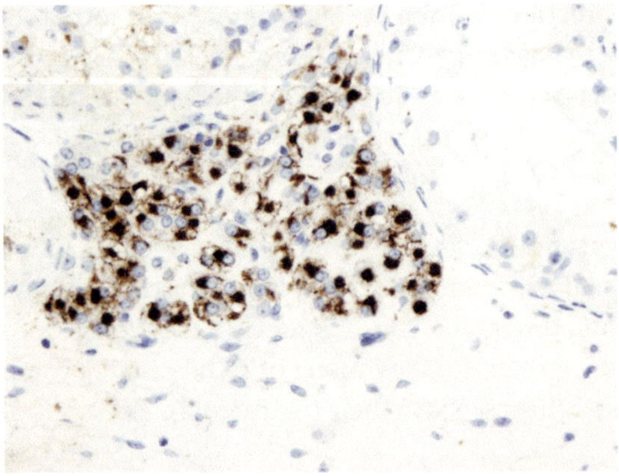

Figure 16. Small-sized Leydig cell cluster showing intense cytoplasmic cytokeratin AE1/AE3 immunostaining in a 75-year-old patient. Autopsy finding.

related to steroidogenesis (e.g., smooth endoplasmic reticulum, mitochondria) [55]. Most of the alterations correspond to those of a primary hypogonadism [56, 57].

7.2.2. Secondary alterations

The most well-known secondary changes are secondary to an obstruction, ischemia, multiple transfusions, acquired hypogonadotropic hypogonadism, and estrogen treatment. When the blockage occurs near the testicle, the seminiferous tubules of several lobules first dilate and later lose the seminiferous epithelium and become sclerosed. Leydig cells acquire a pseudohyperplastic appearance. When a branch of the testicular artery develops arteritis or even partial obstruction by arteriosclerosis, the seminiferous tubules atrophy and the Leydig cells disappear [58]. This image contrasts with the conservation of the surrounding parenchyma. In patients with chronic anemia who undergo multiple transfusions, iron accumulates in the cytoplasm of Leydig cells. In acquired hypogonadotropic hypogonadism, an involution of both the seminiferous tubules and the Leydig cells occurs. The seminiferous epithelium is reduced to only dedifferentiated Sertoli cells and isolated spermatogonia. The thickened tubular wall conserves the elastic fibers, and the Leydig cells involute until they disappear. Estrogen treatment was widely used in the past in prostate cancer, although currently it is only used before proceeding to surgical gender change. Parallel with the dedifferentiation of the seminiferous epithelium is a rapid involution of the Leydig cells, which are reduced to small pyknotic cells with retracted nuclei with some cytoplasmic vacuoles [59].

Acknowledgements

The authors are grateful for the financial assistance from Roche Farma SA and Foundation Domingo Martínez.

Conflict of interest

The authors declare no conflict of interest.

Author details

Maria P. De Miguel[1]*, Pilar Gonzalez-Peramato[2] and Manuel Nistal[3]

*Address all correspondence to: mariapdemiguel@gmail.com

1 Cell Engineering Laboratory, La Paz University Hospital Research Institute, IdiPAZ, Madrid, Spain

2 Department of Pathology, La Paz University Hospital, Madrid, Autonomous University of Madrid, Madrid, Spain

3 Department of Anatomy, Histology and Neuroscience, Autonomous University of Madrid, Madrid, Spain

References

[1] Huhtaniemi I, Pelliniemi LJ. Fetal Leydig cells: Cellular origin, morphology, life span, and special functional features. Proceedings of the Society for Experimental Biology and Medicine. 1992;**201**:125-140

[2] Barsoum IB, Kaur J, Ge RS, Cooke PS, Yao HH. Dynamic changes in fetal Leydig cell populations influence adult Leydig cell populations in mice. The FASEB Journal. 2013; **27**:2657-2666

[3] Shima Y, Morohashi KI. Leydig progenitor cells in fetal testis. Molecular and Cellular Endocrinology. 2017;**445**:55-64

[4] Griswold SL, Behringer RR. Fetal Leydig cell origin and development. Sexual Development. 2009;**3**:1-15

[5] Prince FP. The triphasic nature of Leydig cell development in humans, and comments on nomenclature. The Journal of Endocrinology. 2001;**168**:213-216

[6] Habert R, Lejeune H, Saez JM. Origin, differentiation and regulation of fetal and adult Leydig cells. Molecular and Cellular Endocrinology. 2001;**179**:47-74

[7] Kerr JB, Knell CM. The fate of fetal Leydig cells during the development of the fetal and postnatal rat testis. Development. 1988;**103**:535-544

[8] Nistal M, Paniagua R, Regadera J, Santamarìa L, Amat P. A quantitative morphological study of human Leydig cells from birth to adulthood. Cell and Tissue Research. 1986;**246**:229-236

[9] Shima Y, Matsuzaki S, Miyabayashi K, Otake H, Baba T, Kato S, Huhtaniemi I, Morohashi K. Fetal Leydig cells persist as an androgen-independent subpopulation in the postnatal testis. Molecular Endocrinology. 2015;**29**:1581-1593

[10] Nistal M, Paniagua R, González-Peramato P, Reyes-Mugica M. Perspectives in pediatric pathology: Chapter 2. Testicular descent. Pediatric and Developmental Pathology. 2015;**18**:103-108

[11] Kim JW, Bak CW, Chin MU, Cha DH, Yoon TK, Shim SH. SRY-negative 46,XX infertile male with Leydig cell hyperplasia: Clinical, cytogenetic, and molecular analysis and review of the literature. Fertility and Sterility. 2010;**94**:753.e5-753.e9

[12] Saenger P. New developments in congenital lipoid adrenal hyperplasia and steroidogenic acute regulatory protein. Pediatric Clinics of North America. 1997;**44**:397-421

[13] Sapunar J, Vidal T. Bauer K. Abnormalities of adrenal steroidogenesis in Chilean boys with micropenis. Revista Médica de Chile. 2003;**131**:46-54

[14] Dumić M, Plavsić V, Fattorini I, Ille J. Absent spermatogenesis despite early bilateral orchidopexy in 17-ketoreductase deficiency. Hormone Research. 1985;**22**:100-106

[15] Ascoli M, Fanelli F, Segaloff DL. The lutropin/choriogonadotropin receptor, a 2002 perspective. Endocrine Reviews. 2002;**23**:141-174

[16] Themmen APN, Huhtaniemi IT. Mutations of gonadotropins and gonadotropin receptors: Elucidating the physiology and pathophysiology of pituitary-gonadal function. Endocrine Reviews. 2000;**21**:551-583

[17] Kossack N, Troppmann B, Richter-Unruh A, Kleinau G, Gromoll J. Aberrant transcription of the LHCGR gene caused by a mutation in exon 6A leads to Leydig cell hypoplasia type II. Molecular and Cellular Endocrinology. 2013;**366**:59-67

[18] Husmann DA. Testicular descent: A hypothesis and review of current controversies. Pediatric Endocrinology Reviews. 2009;**6**:491-495

[19] Nistal M, González-Peramato P, Paniagua R. Congenital Leydig cell hyperplasia. Histopathology. 1988;**12**:307-317

[20] Codesal J1, Regadera J, Nistal M, Regadera-Sejas J, Paniagua R. Involution of human fetal Leydig cells. An immunohistochemical, ultrastructural and quantitative study. Journal of Anatomy. 1990;**172**:103-114

[21] Hadziselimovic F, Zivkovic D, Bica DT, Emmons LR. The importance of mini-puberty for fertility in cryptorchidism. The Journal of Urology. 2005;**174**(4 Pt 2):1536-1539

[22] Kurtoğlu S, Baştuğ O. Mini puberty and its interpretation. Turk Pediatri Arsivi. 2014; **49**:186-191

[23] Camats N, Pandey AV, Fernández-Cancio M, Andaluz P, Janner M, Torán N, Moreno F, Bereket A, Akcay T, García-García E, Muñoz MT, Gracia R, Nistal M, Castaño L, Mullis PE, Carrascosa A, Audí L, Flück CE. Ten novel mutations in the NR5A1 gene cause disordered sex development in 46,XY and ovarian insufficiency in 46,XX individuals. The Journal of Clinical Endocrinology and Metabolism. 2012;**97**:E1294-E1306

[24] Laue L, Chan WY, Hsueh AJ, Kudo M, Hsu SY, Wu SM, Blomberg L, Cutler GB Jr. Genetic heterogeneity of constitutively activating mutations of the human luteinizing hormone receptor in familial male-limited precocious puberty. Proceedings of the National Academy of Sciences of the United States of America. 1995;**92**:1906-1910

[25] Gondos B, Egli CA, Rosenthal SM, Grumbach MM. Testicular changes in gonadotropin-independent familial male sexual precocity. Familial testotoxicosis. Archives of Pathology & Laboratory Medicine. 1985;**109**:990-995

[26] De Luca F, Mitchell V, Wasniewska M, Arrigo T, Messina MF, Valenzise M, de Sanctis L, Lahlou N. Regulation of spermatogenesis in McCune-Albright syndrome: Lessons from a 15-year follow-up. European Journal of Endocrinology. 2008;**158**:921-927

[27] Nair M, Kusumakumary P, Ninan A. Precocious puberty as initial presentation in mediastinal tumour. Indian Pediatrics. 2013;**50**:424-426

[28] Seminara SB, Hayes FJ, Crowley WF Jr. Gonadotropin-releasing hormone deficiency in the human (idiopathic hypogonadotropic hypogonadism and Kallmann's syndrome): Pathophysiological and genetic considerations. Endocrine Reviews. 1998;**19**:521-539

[29] Paniagua R, Rodríguez MC, Nistal M, Fraile B, Regadera J, Amat P. Changes in surface area and number of Leydig cells in relation to the 6 stages of the cycle of the human seminiferous epithelium. Anatomy and Embryology. 1988;**178**:423-427

[30] Svechnikov K, Landreh L, Weisser J, Izzo G, Colón E, Svechnikova I, Söder O. Origin, development and regulation of human Leydig cells. Hormone Research in Pædiatrics. 2010;**73**:93-101

[31] Amat P, Paniagua R, Nistal M, Martín A. Mitosis in adult human Leydig cells. Cell and Tissue Research. 1986;**243**:219-221

[32] Maestre de San Juan A. Teratologia: Falta total de nervios olfatorios con anosmia en un individuo en quien existía una atrofia congénita de los testículos y miembro viril. El Siglo Médico. 1856;**131**:211-221

[33] Nistal M, Paniagua R, González-Peramato P, Reyes-Múgica M. Perspectives in pediatric pathology, chapter 18. Hypogonadotropic hypogonadisms. Pediatric and pubertal presentations. Pediatric and Developmental Pathology. 2016;**19**:291-309

[34] Nistal M, González-Peramato P, Serrano A. Chap. 20. Fertility potential of patients with hypogonadotropic hypogonadism. In: Clues in the Diagnosis of Non-tumoral Testicular Pathology. Cham, Switzerland: Springer; 2017. pp. 166-170

[35] Valdés Socin H, Beckers A. Pasqualini's syndrome: Hypoandrogenism with spermatogenesisMedicina (B Aires). 2015;**75**:53-58

[36] Juul A, Almstrup K, Andersson AM, Jensen TK, Jørgensen N, Main KM, Rajpert-De Meyts E, Toppari J, Skakkebæk NE. Possible fetal determinants of male infertility. Nature Reviews. Endocrinology. 2014;**10**:553-562

[37] Soerensen RR, Johannsen TH, Skakkebaek NE, Rajpert-De Meyts E. Leydig cell clustering and Reinke crystal distribution in relation to hormonal function in adult patients

with testicular dysgenesis syndrome (TDS) including cryptorchidism. Hormones (Athens, Greece). 2016;**15**:518-526

[38] Nistal M, Paniagua R, González-Peramato P, Reyes-Múgica M. Perspectives in pediatric pathology, Chapter 6. Male undermasculinization. Pediatric and Developmental Pathology. 2015;**18**:279-296

[39] Abou Alchamat G, Madania A, Alhalabi M. Mild androgen insensitivity syndrome (MAIS): The identification of c.1783C>T mutation in two unrelated infertile men. BML Case Reports. 2017. pii: bcr-2017-220361

[40] Nistal M, Santamaria L, Paniagua R. Quantitative and ultrastructural study of Leydig cells in Klinefelter's syndrome. The Journal of Pathology. 1985;**146**:323-331

[41] Paniagua R, Nistal M, Bravo MP. Leydig cell types in primary testicular disorders. Human Pathology. 1984;**15**:181-190

[42] Nistal M, Paniagua R, López-Pajares I. Ultrastructure of Leydig cells in Klinefelter's syndrome with 48, XXYY karyotype. Virchows Archiv. B: Cell Pathology. 1978;**28**:39-46

[43] Nistal M, Paniagua R. Ultrastructure of testicular biopsy from an XX male. Virchows Archiv. B, Cell Pathology Including Molecular Pathology. 1979;**31**:45-55

[44] Libber SM, Migeon CJ, Brown FR 3rd, Moser HW. Adrenal and testicular function in 14 patients with adrenoleukodystrophy or adrenomyeloneuropathy. Hormone Research. 1986;**24**(1):1-8

[45] Wang X, Stocco DM. The decline in testosterone biosynthesis during male aging: A consequence of multiple alterations. Molecular and Cellular Endocrinology. 2005;**238**:1-7

[46] Yeap BB, Almeida OP, Hyde Z, Norman PE, Chubb SA, Jamrozik K, Flicker L. In men older than 70 years, total testosterone remains stable while free testosterone declines with age. The Health in Men Study. European Journal of Endocrinology. 2007;**156**:585-594

[47] Tajar A, Huhtaniemi IT, O'Neill TW, Finn JD, Pye SR, Lee DM, Bartfai G, Boonen S, Casanueva FF, Forti G, Giwercman A, Han TS, Kula K, Labrie F, Lean ME, Pendleton N, Punab M, Vanderschueren D, Wu FC, EMAS Group. Characteristics of androgen deficiency in late-onset hypogonadism: Results from the European Male Aging Study (EMAS). The Journal of Clinical Endocrinology and Metabolism. 2012;**97**:1508-1516

[48] Gunes S, Hekim GN, Arslan MA, Asci R. Effects of aging on the male reproductive system. Journal of Assisted Reproduction and Genetics. 2016;**33**:441-454

[49] Kothari LK, Gupta AS. Effect of ageing on the volume, structure and total Leydig cell content of the human testis. International Journal of Fertility. 1974;**19**:140-146

[50] Kaler LW, Neaves WB. Attrition of the human Leydig cell population with advancing age. The Anatomical Record. 1978;**192**:513-518

[51] Mori H, Hiromoto N, Nakahara M, Shiraishi T. Stereological analysis of Leydig cell ultrastructure in aged humans. The Journal of Clinical Endocrinology and Metabolism. 1982;**55**:634-641

[52] Nistal M, Santamaria L, Paniagua R, Regadera J, Codesal J. Multinucleate Leydig cells in normal human testes. Andrologia. 1986;**18**:268-272

[53] Paniagua R, Nistal M, Sáez FJ, Fraile B. Ultrastructure of the aging human testis. Journal of Electron Microscopy Technique. 1991;**19**:241-260

[54] Paniagua R, Amat P, Nistal M, Martin A. Ultrastructure of Leydig cells in human ageing testes. Journal of Anatomy. 1986;**146**:173-183

[55] Regadera J, Cobo P, Martínez-García F, Nistal M, Paniagua R. Testosterone immunoexpression in human Leydig cells of the tunica albuginea testis and spermatic cord. A quantitative study in normal foetuses, young adults, elderly men and patients with cryptorchidism. Andrologia. 1993;**25**:115-122

[56] Neaves WB, Johnson L, Porter JC, Parker CR Jr, Petty CS. Leydig cell numbers, daily sperm production, and serum gonadotropin levels in aging men. The Journal of Clinical Endocrinology and Metabolism. 1984;**59**:756-763

[57] Paniagua R, Martín A, Nistal M, Amat P. Testicular involution in elderly men: Comparison of histologic quantitative studies with hormone patterns. Fertility and Sterility. 1987;**47**:671-679

[58] Regadera J, Nistal M, Paniagua R. Testis, epididymis, and spermatic cord in elderly men. Correlation of angiographic and histologic studies with systemic arteriosclerosis. Archives of Pathology & Laboratory Medicine. 1985;**109**:663-667

[59] Nistal M, Gonzalez-Peramato P, De Miguel MP. Sertoli cell dedifferentiation in human cryptorchidism and gender reassignment shows similarities between fetal environmental and adult medical treatment estrogen and antiandrogen exposure. Reproductive Toxicology. 2013;**42**:172-179

Chapter 2

The Regulation of the Male Hypothalamic-Pituitary-Gonadal Axis and Testosterone Production by Adipokines

Alexander O. Shpakov, Julian R. Ryzhov,
Andrey A. Bakhtyukov and Kira V. Derkach

Additional information is available at the end of the chapter

http://dx.doi.org/10.5772/intechopen.76321

Abstract

There is evidence that the mass and metabolic status of the adipose tissue that produces adipokines significantly affect the activity of the hypothalamic-pituitary-gonadal (HPG) axis and the synthesis of testosterone. This is due to the fact that adipokines, such as leptin, adiponectin, visfatin and resistin have an important role in the regulation of the male HPG axis and steroidogenesis in the testes. The regulation of the HPG axis by adipokines can be carried out both through the changes the plasma levels of adipokines (a systemic regulation) and through the changes in the expression and activity of adipokines in the pituitary and testes, the components of the HPG axis (an autonomous regulation). This review presents the comprehensive analysis of the involvement of leptin, adiponectin, resistin and visfatin in the regulation of the male HPG axis and the testosterone production, as well as of the possible mechanisms of this regulation. The role of adipokines in the dysregulation of the male reproductive system and the impaired steroidogenic activity in the testes in obesity and type 2 diabetes mellitus are also discussed.

Keywords: adipokines, testosterone, leptin, hypothalamic-pituitary-gonadal axis, obesity

1. Introduction

There is much evidence that significant changes in the body and fat weight in men with metabolic disorders, such as severe obesity and type 2 diabetes mellitus (DM2), and with long-term fasting can lead to the alteration in the hypothalamic-pituitary-gonadal (HPG) axis, as illustrated by the changed secretion of gonadotropin-releasing hormone (GnRH) and gonadotropins, the reduced testosterone (T) production by Leydig cells and the impaired spermatogenesis. The alterations in the HPG axis, as a result, lead to infertility [1–3]. The relationship between the fat content and androgens level has been demonstrated in animals with obesity and DM2, as well as in fasting conditions [4–6]. All this indicates that adipocyte-produced factors can play an important role in controlling the HPG axis and in regulating the steroidogenesis in Leydig cells. Among these factors, the most interesting are adipokines, such as leptin, adiponectin, resistin and visfatin [3, 7, 8]. It is well known that in metabolic disorders, the plasma levels of these adipokines and the functional activity of adipokines-regulated signaling systems in the target tissues undergo significant changes, which can be considered to be one of the key causes of abnormalities in the HPG axis and androgen deficiency [9–11].

There is evidence that adipokines affect the different components of the male HPG axis. Transferred to the brain through the blood-brain barrier (BBB), adipokines act on the activity of hypothalamic GnRH-expressing neurons, thus changing the GnRH-stimulated production of luteinizing hormone (LH), the main regulator of T synthesis, by pituitary gonadotrophs [12, 13]. The adipokines can directly affect the gonadotrophs producing LH, and in this regulation both the adipokines circulating in the bloodstream and the adipokines synthesized within the pituitary can be involved [14, 15]. Some adipokines can also directly affect the functions of Leydig cells, as indicated by a high level of adipokines expression in the testes, as well as detection of the main components of the adipokine signaling, including adipokine-specific receptors, in testicular cells, including Leydig cells [16–19]. The study of the effects of leptin, adiponectin and other adipokines on the male HPG axis and their role in the regulation of steroidogenesis is a major problem of clinical endocrinology and reproductive medicine. The solution of this problem will allow developing the new approaches for restoring the reproductive functions and androgen status in men with endocrine and metabolic disorders, which is based on the normalization of the adipokine signaling in the CNS and at the periphery.

This review presents the comprehensive analysis of the involvement of leptin, adiponectin, resistin and visfatin in the regulation of the male HPG axis and steroidogenesis, as well as of the possible mechanisms of this regulation. The role of adipokines in the dysregulation of the male reproductive system and the impaired steroidogenic activity in the testes in obesity and DM2 are also discussed.

2. Leptin

2.1. Leptin and its signaling system

Leptin, a 167-amino acid polypeptide hormone encoded by the *ob* gene, is produced preferably by the adipose tissue and is involved in the regulation of eating behavior, energy expenditure and endocrine functions [20–22]. Fasting reduces the plasma leptin level, while food intake, on the contrary, leads to its elevation. A prolonged increase in the plasma leptin level leads to leptin resistance, resulting in the impaired metabolism and eating behavior [23, 24]. Along with the adipose tissue, the *ob* gene expression is detected in other tissues, including the pituitary and testes [25].

The regulatory effects of leptin are realized due to its specific interaction with leptin receptors (Ob-R) that are generated by alternative splicing and include at least six isoforms [26]. The full-length isoform Ob-Rb is active and expressed in the hypothalamus with high intensity [27, 28]. The truncated isoforms, Ob-Ra, Ob-Rc, Ob-Rd and Ob-Rf are inactive, but retain the ability to bind to leptin at its excess. It is assumed that they carry out the receptor-mediated transport of leptin through the BBB and, possibly, through other tissue barriers [29, 30]. In the arcuate nuclei (ARC) of hypothalamus, leptin binds to Ob-Rb receptor, which leads to the phosphorylation of JAK2, a non-receptor tyrosine kinase, that phosphorylates the Tyr^{985}, Tyr^{1077} and Tyr^{1138} residues located within the intracellular domain of Ob-Rb, each responsible for the activation of certain signaling cascade [23]. It has been shown that the phospho-Tyr^{985} is responsible for activation of Src Homology 2 domain-containing protein tyrosine phosphatase 2 (SHP-2) and the mitogen-activated protein kinases (MAPK), such as extracellular signal-related kinases-1/2 (ERK1/2), c-Jun amino-terminal kinases (JNK) and p38-MAPK, which are involved in the regulation of cell growth and differentiation. The targets of MAPK are different transcription factors, including c-Fos, c-Jun and cAMP response element-binding protein (CREB), which control the expression of a large number of genes [3, 31]. The phospho-Tyr^{1138} is responsible for activation of the transcription factor STAT3 (signal transducer and activator of transcription-3) regulating the expression of genes involved in metabolic and growth processes. In turn, phospho-Tyr^{1077} induces the activation of the transcription factor STAT5, responsible for the regulation of energy metabolism and endocrine system [23, 32].

Another mechanism of leptin action is the activation of 3-phosphoinositide pathway, which involves phosphatidylinositol-3-kinase (PI3K) and Akt kinase controlling the activity of the multi-component kinase mTOR complex 1. Since Akt-mediated inhibition of this complex in the hypothalamic ARC leads to a decrease in the expression of the *Kiss1* gene encoding polypeptide kisspeptin, there is reason to believe that the mTOR complex 1 is involved in the regulation of hypothalamic kisspeptin signaling [33]. The leptin-induced activation of the kisspeptin/neurokinin B/dynorphin (KNDy)-neurons leads to the secretion of kisspeptin that triggers the GnRH secretion by the GnRH-expressing neurons, the main target of kisspeptin [34, 35]. The other targets of Akt kinase are the transcription factors Nur77 and CREB that are involved in the regulation of the reproduction. Along with the 3-phosphoinositide pathway, leptin activates AMP-activated protein kinase (AMPK), the most important energy sensor of the cells, and stimulates protein phosphotyrosine phosphatase 1B and the suppressor of cytokine signaling 3 (SOCS3), the negative regulators of the leptin signaling that are responsible for leptin resistance [23, 36].

2.2. The mechanisms of leptin action on the male reproductive system and testosterone synthesis

In the recent years, the evidence has been obtained that leptin plays a very important role in the control of male reproductive functions and puberty, which is based on leptin-mediated regulation of the HPG axis [8, 37]. The *ob/ob* double knockout male mice had severe obesity, metabolic and hormonal abnormalities, and were infertile. A low-fat diet led to a decrease in the body and fat weight, but did not allow recovery of fertility in the *ob/ob* mice [38, 39]. The administration of leptin to *ob/ob* male mice, along with the improved energy expenditure and metabolic processes, led to the onset of puberty and partially restored reproductive functions, which was due to the normalization of the GnRH and gonadotropins secretion [4, 8, 37]. In the prepubertal period, the mutations in the *ob* gene, along with the early obesity, lead to the reduced levels of LH and follicle-stimulating hormone (FSH) and induce the signs of hypogonadotropic hypogonadism and the impaired reproductive functions [40–43].

A survey of men from Slovenia, Macedonia and Serbia with three different mononucleotide mutations within the *ob* gene showed that infertility was characteristic for men with only a polymorphism rs10244329 [42]. The polymorphism 2548G/A (genotype AA) in the *ob* gene in Iranian men was also associated with reproductive dysfunctions. However, the polymorphism with the genotype AG was much more common in men with normal fertility, which can indicate its protective effect on the male reproductive system [43].

The mutations within the *Ob-R* gene had a less pronounced effect on the male reproduction, which was illustrated by the experimental and clinical studies. The polymorphisms in this gene, as a rule, had a little influence on the male reproductive system and did not cause infertility [42, 43]. As in the *ob/ob* mice, the delayed puberty was shown in the *db/db* double knockout male mice lacking a functionally active receptor Ob-Rb, but the animals retained fertility [37]. Unlike men, women with inactivating mutations in the *Ob-R* gene had the pronounced reproductive dysfunctions and the decreased levels of estradiol, gonadotropins and GnRH [44, 45].

The effects of leptin on the male HPG axis can be carried out at the level of hypothalamic neurons, pituitary gonadotrophs and testicular cells. It is important to note that the response of the HPG axis to leptin depends on the dose of this adipokine and the duration of treatment, the metabolic and hormonal status, as well as the functional state of the leptin signaling system in the target tissues. This is well illustrated by the data on the influence of leptin on the hypothalamic structures. It is shown that a single i.c.v. administration of leptin to ovariectomized female rats under starvation conditions, when the leptin level was reduced, led to a rapid increase in the plasma LH level, which demonstrates leptin-mediated stimulation of secretory activity of the GnRH-neurons [12, 46]. At the same time, under conditions of prolonged administration of leptin, an increase in LH level [47] or lack of leptin effect on LH secretion [48] were detected, which may be assumed to be due to varying degrees of leptin resistance in the case of long-term action of leptin on hypothalamic neurons. This was supported by the fact that the action of low, nanomolar concentrations of leptin on the ARC and the ventromedial nuclei of the hypothalamus led to an increase in the GnRH secretion, while high, micromolar leptin concentrations did not cause this effect [5, 37]. The i.c.v. administration of leptin to fasting cows led to an increase of both basal and GnRH-stimulated LH secretion, while the administration of leptin to fed animals with the increased leptin level did not induce significant changes in LH level [49, 50]. Thus, the stimulating effect of leptin on the HPG axis at the hypothalamic level was largely dependent on eating behavior, and was the main mechanism that mediates the relationship between the satiety and metabolic status, on the one hand, and the gonadotropins levels and activity of the steroidogenesis system, on the other.

2.2.1. Hypothalamus

The central effects of leptin on the HPG axis are mediated through its interaction with leptin receptors located on hypothalamic ARC neurons expressing either pro-opiomelanocortin

http://dx.doi.org/10.5772/intechopen.76321

(POMC) or agouti-related peptide (AgRP) and neuropeptide Y (NPY). Due to activation of these neurons by leptin, the positive (POMC-neurons) or negative (AgRP/NPY-neurons) regulation of GnRH-neurons occurs, especially since these neurons themselves do not contain the receptor Ob-Rb and, therefore, can not be target for leptin (**Figure 1**).

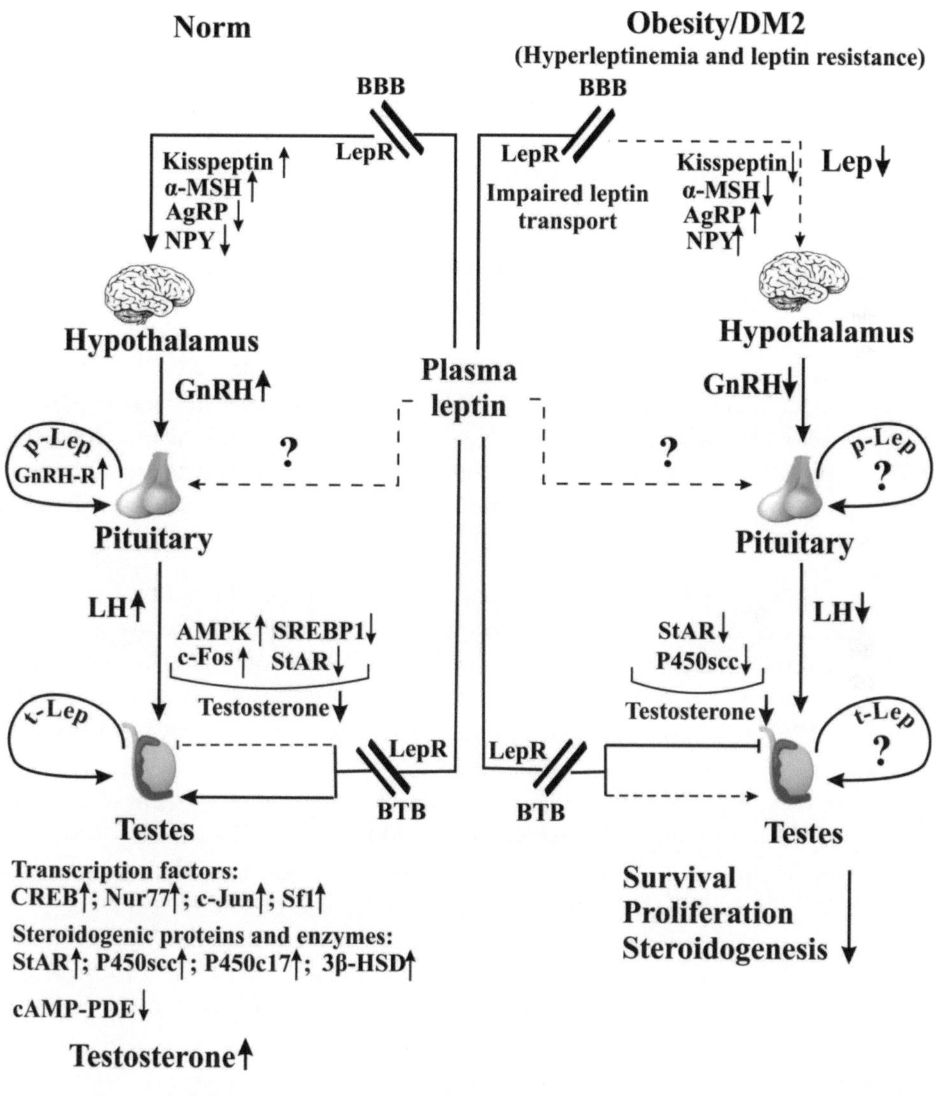

Figure 1. The regulatory effects of the plasma, pituitary and testicular leptin on the male HPG axis and the testosterone synthesis in the testes in the norm and in the metabolic disorders. Abbreviations: p-Lep and t-Lep, the pituitary and testicular leptin; LepR, leptin receptor; GnRH, gonadotropin-releasing hormone; GnRH-R, receptor of GnRH; LH, luteinizing hormone; T, testosterone; AMPK, AMP-activated protein kinase; CREB, cAMP response element-binding protein; Nur77, c-Jun, c-Fos and Sf1, transcription factors Nur77, c-Jun, c-Fos and Sf1; SREBP1, sterol regulatory element-binding protein-1; cAMP-PDE, cAMP-specific phosphodiesterase; StAR, steroidogenic acute regulatory protein; P450scc and P450c17, cytochromes $P450_{scc}$ (P450 cholesterol side chain cleavage enzyme) and P450c17; 3β-HSD, 3β-hydroxysteroid dehydrogenase; α-MSH, α-melanocyte-stimulating hormone; AgRP, agouti-related peptide; NPY, neuropeptide Y; BBB, blood-brain barrier; BTB, blood-testicular barrier.

Leptin-induced activation of ObRb located on the POMC-neurons leads to an increase in the production of POMC-derived melanocortin peptides, primarily α-melanocyte-stimulating hormone (α-MSH), an agonist of types 3 and 4 melanocortin receptors (MC_3R and MC_4R) [51]. The α-MSH binds to $MC_{3/4}R$ located on GnRH-neurons, and stimulates the GnRH secretion by them. In favor of this mechanism, there is evidence that the administration of leptin to the preoptic area of the hypothalamus leads simultaneously to an increase in α-MSH level and a stimulation of GnRH secretion [52]. The $MC_{3/4}R$ agonists, such as α-MSH and its analogue melanotan-II are also effective, increasing GnRH release [53, 54]. It should be noted that at least 70% of GnRH-neurons are activated by α-MSH [53]. Both MC_3R and MC_4R are involved in the effects of melanocortin peptides on GnRH-neurons, since mice lacking only one type of MCR remain capable of reproduction [55, 56].

Another mechanism for leptin regulation of GnRH secretion, in which the melanocortin peptides also participate, is more complex. In accordance with this, in the first stage the melanocortin peptides secreted by POMC-neurons interact with MCR located on the KNDy-neurons. Kisspeptin released from KNDy-neurons binds to the kisspeptin receptors located on GnRH-neurons and stimulates GnRH secretion [57]. In the hypothalamic ARC, the outgrowths of POMC-neurons form the contacts with the bodies of KNDy-neurons, and a release of α-MSH by POMC-neurons causes a rapid depolarization of KNDy-neurons. Pharmacological inhibition of MC_3R and MC_4R by the antagonist SHU9119 decreases the expression of kisspeptin by 45%. The stimulating effect of melanotan-II on LH production in mice lacking the kisspeptin receptor GPR54 was reduced significantly [57].

The AgRP, the endogenous $MC_{3/4}R$ antagonist, and NPY, both produced by the AgRP/NPY-neurons, mediate the inhibitory effect of leptin on LH production by pituitary gonadotrophs. However, the degradation of AgRP/NPY-neurons and the knockout of the *Ob-R* gene in them, making these neurons insensitive to leptin, lead to a delay in puberty in mice and reduce their fertility [58, 59]. The most important in the regulation of reproductive functions is NPY, which, by binding to the receptors Y1 and Y5 on the GnRH-neurons [60], suppresses GnRH expression and lowers the plasma LH levels [61, 62]. A prolonged treatment of animals with NPY suppresses the production of gonadotropins and terminates the puberty [63, 64]. Leptin suppresses NPY expression, preventing its inhibitory effect on the HPG axis. Insulin also inhibits NPY expression [63]. The similarity of the leptin and insulin effects on NPY expression is due to the fact that the main target for leptin and insulin is the 3-phosphoinositide cascade, which is believed to be involved in positive regulation of POMC production and in negative regulation of NPY and AgRP production within the ARC [65, 66].

2.2.2. Pituitary

Leptin can stimulate LH production, acting directly on gonadotrophs (**Figure 1**). Unlike the hypothalamus, where leptin is mainly transferred from the bloodstream, its source in gonadotrophs can be either the plasma leptin or pituitary leptin synthesized by gonadotrophs [67, 68]. There is a good reason to believe that pituitary leptin functions as a paracrine and autocrine regulator controlling the survival and functional activity of gonadotrophs, since the plasma leptin can not mediate the complex pattern of pituitary hormone secretion [69]. This assumption is supported by the data obtained in mice with tissue-specific knockout of the *ob* gene, either in

http://dx.doi.org/10.5772/intechopen.76321

the adipose tissue or in the pituitary. Mice lacking the *ob* gene in the adipose tissue did not have leptin circulating in the bloodstream. At the same time, they had functionally active somatotrophs, which, like gonadotrophs, are targets for leptin and contain Ob-Rb, as well as normal expression of growth hormone in them. Meanwhile, the plasma level of growth hormone and the expression of growth hormone receptors in the hypothalamus were decreased, which indicates an impairment of the somatotropic axis. The production of leptin in the pituitary cells did not lead to its transfer from the pituitary to the bloodstream, indicating the autonomous function of leptin in the pituitary [70]. These data suggest that for normal hypothalamic-pituitary regulation, both the levels of plasma leptin and the pituitary production of leptin are important, and pituitary leptin is mainly involved in the regulation of survival and secretory activity of pituitary cells, but does not influence significantly the other leptin targets in organism.

The functions of the autonomous leptin system in the pituitary, its participation in gonadotropins production and the relationship between the activity of this system and the physiological state of the HPG axis are supported by the following facts. The *ob* gene is expressed in gonadotrophs, although the data on the number of pituitary cells that produce leptin and on the co-expression of leptin and pituitary hormones differ significantly [15, 71, 72]. In adult males and females, the *ob* gene is expressed in 30% of gonadotrophs [72]. In rats the pituitary leptin level varies significantly during the postnatal development, and in female rats it changes at the different stages of the estrous cycle and during pregnancy [15]. It is shown that leptin influences the production of gonadotropins, changing the GnRH receptor activity and, thereby, controlling the sensitivity of gonadotrophs to hypothalamic regulation [73]. The gene *Ob-R* encoding leptin receptor is expressed in a large number of gonadotrophs, and this suggests that these cells are the main target for leptin [8, 37, 67, 68, 74]. The sensitivity of gonadotrophs to leptin is indicated by the fact that this adipokine at relatively low concentrations, 10^{-9} and 10^{-11} M, stimulates the LH and FSH secretion in the hemi-anterior pituitaries of adult male rats. At the same time, in the *in vivo* conditions, leptin increases LH level, but does not affect the secretion of FSH [46]. The expression of pituitary leptin is controlled by steroid hormones, GnRH and other factors. GnRH and NPY increase the leptin expression by pituitary gonadotrophs, while the gastrointestinal hormone ghrelin, the regulator of food intake and the functional antagonist of leptin, on the contrary, suppresses the *ob* gene expression [69, 72].

2.2.3. Testes

Currently, there is evidence that leptin not only indirectly affects the steroidogenesis in Leydig cells through the regulation of the HPG axis but is also capable of directly affecting the activity of steroidogenesis system [3, 8]. The following facts support this: (1) the transport of leptin circulating in the bloodstream through the blood-testicular barrier (BTB) and the synthesis of leptin in the testicular cells; (2) the expression of leptin receptors and the presence of effector components of the leptin signaling in Leydig cells and (3) the results of the *in vitro* experiments demonstrating the leptin effect on steroidogenesis in the cultured Leydig cells.

In 1999, Banks and coauthors showed that leptin circulating in the blood was transported through the BTB, and the permeability was higher than in the case of the BBB [75]. Based on high rate of leptin transport through the BTB and high permeability of this barrier to other proteins, it was concluded that the mechanisms of leptin transport through the BBB and BTB differ significantly. However, taking into account the high density of the truncated isoform Ob-Ra of leptin receptor on the surface of endothelial cells forming the BTB, there is reason to believe that, like the BBB, leptin transport through the BTB is also a receptor-dependent [37]. In this case, one should expect its dependence on the activity of the leptin signaling system at the periphery and its decrease in the conditions of leptin resistance. Another source of intra-testicular leptin was its synthesis in the testes of adult men and animals. The highest level of the *ob* gene expression was shown in the seminiferous tubules, spermatocytes and spermatozoa [18, 76–79]. In Leydig cells, leptin expression was demonstrated only in pigs [18]. Along with the truncated isoform Ob-Ra, which may be involved in leptin transport through the BTB, a functionally active isoform Ob-Rb was detected in the plasma membrane of testicular cells, preferably Leydig cells, which convincingly demonstrates that activity of these cells is regulated by leptin [37, 80]. It should be noted that in adult men, Ob-Rb is expressed only in Leydig cells [78]. The leptin receptors, although to varying degrees, are expressed in the testes throughout the ontogenesis, including the late embryogenesis [76, 77, 80]. The maximal expression of leptin receptors is observed during the puberty of rats at the age of 1–3 months, which positively correlates with the increased T production.

The effectors, whose activity is regulated by leptin through the activated forms of Ob-Rb and JAK2, control the activity of the transcription factors regulating the expression of steroidogenesis genes in different ways [3]. Leptin-induced stimulation of Akt-kinase and MAPK results in the phosphorylation and activation of the transcription factor CREB that is also activated by gonadotropins via cAMP-dependent pathways [81]. The activation of p38-MAPK and JNK leads to the stimulation of the transcription factors Nur77 and c-Jun [82, 83]. The main targets for these factors are the genes encoding StAR protein responsible for transport of cholesterol into the mitochondria and P450 cholesterol side chain cleavage enzyme (cytochrome $P450_{scc}$) converting cholesterol to pregnenolone [84] (**Figure 1**). Along with this, the activation of MAPK cascade results in an increase in the expression of Sf-1 factor, the coactivator of expression of the gene encoding StAR and the genes *Cyp11a1*, *Cyp17a1* and *Hsd3b1* encoding the steroidogenesis enzymes, cytochromes $P450_{scc}$ and P450c17 and 3β-hydroxysteroid dehydrogenase (3β-HSD) [85–88]. Since the transcription factors Sf-1, CREB, Nur77 and c-Jun are able to enhance steroidogenesis in Leydig cells, the leptin pathways that stimulate their activity are the positive regulators of T production [3].

Leptin activation of the STAT3 and STAT5, as well as leptin-induced ERK1/2-dependent activation of the factor c-Fos lead to the opposite effect and suppress steroidogenesis in Leydig cells. An increase in ERK1/2 activity may be due to the prolonged leptin effect on the system Ob-Rb/JAK2 and, as a result, the activation of SHP-2 phosphatase, which affects the activity of MAPK cascade [89]. A decrease in T production by Leydig cells can be the result of AMPK activation, which suppresses the activity of sterol regulatory element-binding protein-1 (SREBP1) [90]. As is well known, SREBP1 positively regulates the *Star* gene expression [91, 92].

In addition to direct leptin effect on the expression of steroidogenesis genes, this adipokine can modulate the gonadotropin signaling pathways in Leydig cells, inducing an increase in gonadotropin-stimulated T production. It is well known that LH and human chorionic gonadotropin (hCG) specifically bind to LH/hCG receptors located on Leydig cells and stimulate the activity of adenylyl cyclase catalyzing cAMP synthesis, which leads to the activation of protein kinase A and CREB. Further, the level of intracellular cAMP is reduced due to its hydrolysis by cAMP-specific phosphodiesterases (cAMP-PDE), which leads to the attenuation of signal transduction generated by gonadotropins and inhibits their stimulating effect on steroidogenesis. Leptin suppresses the cAMP-PDE activity, maintaining the increased level of intracellular cAMP and thereby potentiates steroidogenic effect of gonadotropins (**Figure 1**). This is supported by the data that leptin enhances the stimulating effect of hCG on the cAMP level in rat Leydig cells [77].

Along with the regulation of T synthesis in Leydig cells, leptin controls the mass and size of the testes, diameter of the seminiferous tubules and spermatogenesis and affects the survival of Leydig cells and other testicular cells [26, 93]. Leptin also regulates steroidogenesis in the ovaries and adrenal glands, and the mechanisms of its regulatory effect are believed to be similar to those in Leydig cells [37, 94].

2.3. Leptin regulation of the male gonadal axis and steroidogenesis in metabolic disorders

In men with obesity, metabolic syndrome and DM2, the activity of the male HPG axis and the T production are decreased, which lead to androgen deficiency [95–97]. Along with this, in diabetic men the plasma level of estrogens and the ratio of estrogen/T are significantly increased, which due to the increased activity of aromatase and the altered production of sex hormone-binding globulin [98–101]. The elevated concentrations of reactive oxygen species and inflammatory factors lead to the damage in Leydig cells and reduce their steroidogenic activity [97, 102].

In obesity and DM2, the plasma leptin level is significantly increased [103, 104], which leads to leptin resistance. As a result, the receptor-mediated transport of leptin through the BBB is reduced, which leads to a decrease in the intrahypothalamic leptin level and to a weakening of the regulatory effects of leptin on hypothalamic neurons and GnRH secretion (**Figure 1**). It is also not possible to exclude the possibility of reducing leptin transport through the BTB, although such data have not yet been obtained.

The detailed study of the relationships between the leptin signaling and androgen deficiency in men with obesity and DM2 are not currently available. In rats with diet-induced obesity, severe hyperleptinemia and leptin resistance was associated with a decrease in the number of Leydig cells by 30%. This can be caused by the reduced intratesticular levels of leptin or the decreased sensitivity of testicular cells to this adipokine that participates in the regulation of survival and proliferation of Leydig cells (**Figure 1**). Although the plasma T level in obese male rats did not change, in the testes of animals it decreased by 25%, which was associated with a decrease in the expression of the *Star* and *Cyp11a1* genes encoding StAR and cytochrome $P450_{scc}$ [105].

The deterioration of reproductive functions was found in mice with a knockout of the gene encoding the catalytic p110α-subunit of PI3K in the adipose tissue [106]. In the testes of 30-day knockout mice with severe hyperleptinemia, the expression of the gene encoding leptin was increased, while the expression of the genes encoding StAR and $P450_{scc}$ was reduced. Adult knockout mice had a severe form of hyperleptinemia, obesity, hepatic steatosis and the impaired glucose tolerance, and were infertile. It was quite unexpected that in the testes of knockout animals the expression of the *ob* gene and the *Hsd17b3* gene encoding 17β-hydroxysteroid dehydrogenase 3 (17β-HSD) was significantly increased, and the plasma level of T was also increased, indicating a pronounced hyperandrogenemia [106]. A possible cause for this was the reduced activity of estrogen receptor-α (Esr1), since in animals lacking the *Esr1* gene a similar phenotype with hyperandrogenemia and infertility was described [107, 108].

3. Adiponectin

3.1. Adiponectin and its signaling system

Polypeptide hormone adiponectin is produced mainly by the adipose tissue [109, 110], but despite this, the plasma adiponectin level is negatively correlated with the body mass index and the reserves of adipose tissue [111]. The plasma level of adiponectin is characterized by gender specificity and significantly lowers in males, which is true for humans and rodents [112]. Adiponectin can be synthesized not only by the adipose tissue but also by the brain, pituitary, testes and others [17, 113]. Adiponectin is consists of a variable N-terminal domain, a large globular C-terminal domain and a collagenous domain located between them, containing 22 collagenous Gly-XY repeats [114–116]. Using the collagenous repeats, adiponectin molecules interact with each other to form the homotrimeric complexes that aggregate into the hexamers and high-molecular complexes similar to those in the case of tumor necrosis factor-α (TNF-α) [117]. To form the trimeric complex, hydroxylation of the proline and lysine residues in the collagenous repeats is necessary, since the lack of this modification does not allow the formation of such complex and leads to a loss in the adiponectin activity [118, 119]. High-molecular complexes of adiponectin are stabilized by disulfide bonds formed between the trimers [120]. The trimeric, hexameric and high-molecular complexes are present in the bloodstream, while the monomeric forms are found in trace amounts [115, 121–123]. Post-translational modifications of adiponectin and its oligomerization significantly affect the bioavailability, binding characteristics and pattern of specific activity of adiponectin [115, 120, 123–125].

The tissues, the targets of adiponectin, express the adiponectin receptors AdipoR1 and AdipoR2, which bind specifically to various forms of adiponectin with different affinity [111, 125–127]. Despite the fact that both these receptors seven times penetrate the plasma membrane, like classical G protein-coupled receptors, they differ significantly from them in membrane topology, having the extracellular C-terminal domain and the intracellular N-terminal domain. In addition, the adiponectin receptors interact with APPL proteins (adaptor protein, phosphotyrosine interacting with plekstrin-homologous domain and leucine zipper), but not with heterotrimeric G-proteins. The AdipoR1 binds with a high affinity to the truncated globular form of adiponectin and with a low affinity with the oligomeric and high-molecular forms of full-length adiponectin, while AdipoR2 binds with an intermediate affinity to both the full-length and globular forms. The both receptors interact with two isoforms of the APPL proteins, APPL-1 and APPL-2 [128, 129]. The interaction of adiponectin-activated AdipoR1 with APPL-1 leads to the activation of AMPK and the 3-phosphoinositide and MAPK cascades. The APPL-2 forms a complex with APPL-1 and prevents APPL-1-mediated regulations.

When adiponectin binds to AdipoR1, the APPL-1/APPL-2 complex dissociates, resulting in the release of APPL-1 to interact with the downstream effector proteins [116, 130].

3.2. The effect of adiponectin on hypothalamic neurons

Adiponectin is able to control steroidogenic function in the testes directly, acting on Leydig cells, and indirectly, acting on the HPG axis at the hypothalamic and pituitary levels. To interact with hypothalamic neurons, the main target of adiponectin in the CNS, it is necessary to transport adiponectin into the brain through the BBB. It is suggested that the receptor-mediated transport of adiponectin through the BBB can be carried out through the AdipoR1 and AdipoR2 receptors located on the endothelium of cerebral vessels (**Figure 2**). In addition, a large number of adiponectin receptors and the components of adiponectin-regulated signaling pathways have been identified in the ARC and paraventricular nuclei of the hypothalamus [131–134] and in other brain areas [13]. Adiponectin is easily transferred from the bloodstream to the brain and cerebrospinal fluid (CSF), although its concentration in the CSF is low, being only 0.1% of that in the blood [132–135]. In obesity, which was characterized by the reduced plasma level

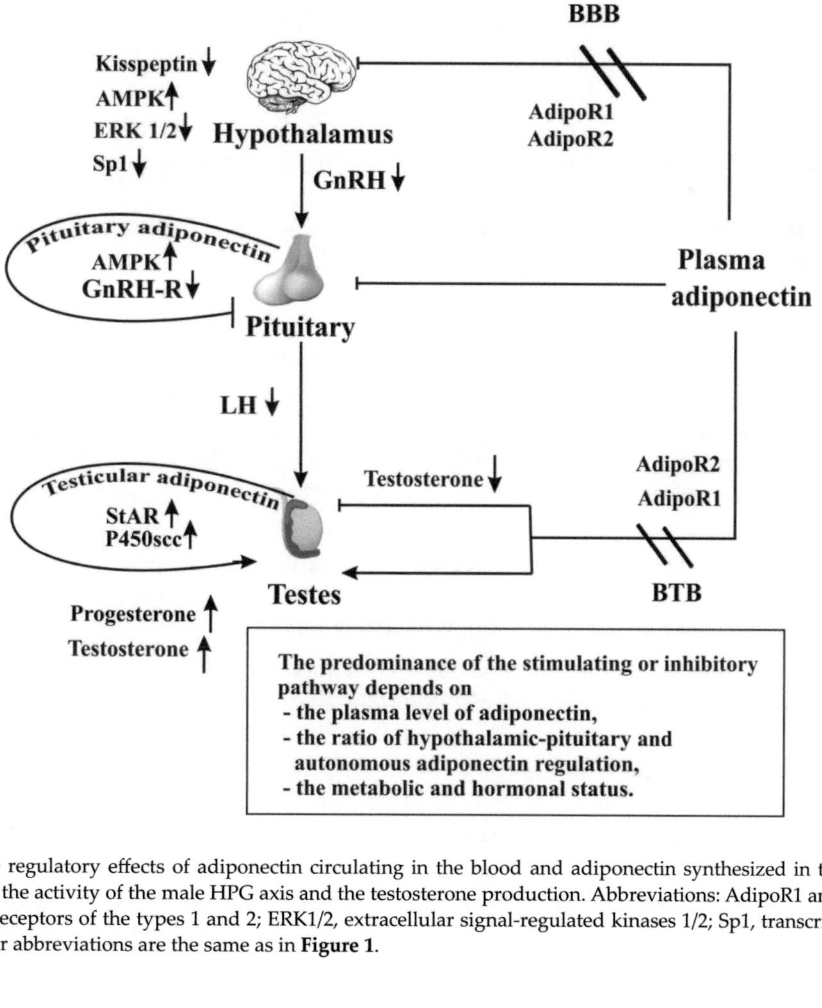

Figure 2. The regulatory effects of adiponectin circulating in the blood and adiponectin synthesized in the pituitary and testes on the activity of the male HPG axis and the testosterone production. Abbreviations: AdipoR1 and AdipoR2, adiponectin receptors of the types 1 and 2; ERK1/2, extracellular signal-regulated kinases 1/2; Sp1, transcription factor Sp1. The other abbreviations are the same as in **Figure 1**.

of adiponectin [134, 136, 137], its concentration in the brain areas was also decreased [134]. It should be noted that, as in the case of circulating adiponectin, a negative correlation was found between the adiponectin level in the CSF and the body mass [133, 134]. Thus, unlike leptin, intracerebral adiponectin deficiency in obesity is caused by a reduced level of this adipokine in the blood. Although there is evidence that adiponectin can be synthesized in the CNS [17, 113], the greatest, if not all, amount of this adipokine comes from the periphery, and the intracerebral level of adiponectin depends on the activity of adiponectin-transporting system of the brain.

Upon binding to adiponectin receptors in neurons of the paraventricular nuclei and the periventricular region of the hypothalamus, adiponectin activates AMPK [13, 138], decreases the activity of ERK1/2 [13], causes a weakening of the calcium-dependent signaling pathways and inhibits the hyperpolarization-activated cationic currents responsible for pacemaker activity of GnRH-neurons [139]. It is important to note that the inhibition of ERK1/2 activity is due to an increase in AMPK activity [13]. The main result of adiponectin action on GnRH-neurons is a decrease in the synthesis and secretion of GnRH and, as a consequence, a decreased LH production by gonadotrophs [13, 139] (**Figure 2**).

Adiponectin also interacts with the KNDy-neurons expressing kisspeptin. Adiponectin-induced increase in AMPK activity in these neurons results in the inhibition of AMPK-dependent transport of the transcription factor SP1 into the nucleus, which is illustrated by SP1 accumulation in the cytoplasm. As a result, the expression of the *KISS1* gene is reduced, which leads to a decrease of the stimulating effect of kisspeptin on the activity of GnRH-neurons [140]. There is reason to believe that a decrease in the SP1 activity may be due to adiponectin-induced inhibition of ERK1/2 activity in the KNDy-neurons [141].

3.3. The effect of adiponectin on pituitary gonadotrophs

The inhibitory effect of adiponectin on LH production can be carried out at the pituitary level, since both adiponectin receptors were detected in the LH-expressing gonadotrophs of human and rats [14, 142, 143]. In addition, the expression of the *Adiponectin* gene was detected in the pituitary gland [142–144], whereby the regulators of the adiponectin receptors in gonadotrophs can be both plasma and pituitary adiponectin (**Figure 2**). A long-term treatment of the primary culture of gonadotrophs with adiponectin results in a decrease in the AdipoR1 expression, but has a little effect on the expression of AdipoR2, indicating the development of receptor-specific resistance of gonadotrophs to adiponectin [144]. Adiponectin inhibits both the basal and GnRH-stimulated LH secretion, and its effect is detected even after a short exposure with gonadotrophs [14, 144]. This is largely due to adiponectin-induced decrease in the expression of GnRH receptors in gonadotrophs [144]. As in the hypothalamic GnRH- and KNDy-neurons, regulatory effects of adiponectin on gonadotrophs are mediated by its ability to activate AMPK [14]. Although adiponectin inhibits LH secretion [14, 138, 144], it has very little effect on FSH secretion [14]. This indicates that the targets of adiponectin in the pituitary are preferably gonadotrophs that produce LH.

3.4. The effect of adiponectin on the testes

As noted above, the expression of the *Adiponectin* gene was found in the testes, which demonstrates the intratesticular production of adiponectin, and the main source of this adipokine is

Leydig cells [17]. Three transcripts of the *Adiponectin* gene, 2.5, 1.8 and 1.2 kb, were detected in the adipose tissue, while in Leydig cells were only two transcripts, 1.2 and <1.0 kb, and in both cases the adiponectin isoform with a molecular weight of 30 kDa was dominant [17]. However, the contribution of the adiponectin synthesized in the testes to total pool of intratesticular adiponectin is difficult to assess, especially since the plasma adiponectin level is significantly higher than in the testes and seminal fluid. The concentration of adiponectin in the seminal fluid of healthy men is 100 times lower than in the bloodstream. The adiponectin level in the semen of men and bulls is positively correlated with its plasma level [145, 146]. Furthermore, adiponectin level in the seminal fluid positively correlates with the number of spermatozoa, their mobility and normal morphology [145]. In men with a vasectomy that excludes the intratesticular sources of adiponectin, this level in the seminal fluid does not change. These facts suggest that the main, if not the only, source of adiponectin in the semen is adiponectin, coming from the bloodstream. On the other hand, the source of adiponectin in Leydig cells can be both plasma and intratesticular adiponectin [116, 123].

The main regulators of the *Adiponectin* gene expression in the testes are gonadotropins with LH activity. The production of adiponectin in the testes of hypophysectomized rats is significantly reduced, but is completely restored after their treatment with hCG. In rats, during the neonatal period, when LH level is low, the content of adiponectin in the testes is also very low. During puberty, when plasma LH concentration and the proliferation of Leydig cells are increased, the expression of adiponectin also increased rapidly, reaching a maximum in rats at 2 months of age [17]. There is a positive correlation between the adiponectin levels and the T production, because the T synthesis also depends on gonadotropins with LH activity [147]. Unlike LH and hCG, FSH has a little effect on the adiponectin content in the testes, which is due to the fact that the expression of adiponectin in the Sertoli cells, the main target for FSH, has not been identified. The expression of adiponectin in the testes is also controlled by thyroid hormones and corticosteroids. An increase in thyroid hormone levels due to therapy with L-thyroxine causes an increase in the *Adiponectin* gene expression, while the treatment with dexamethasone leads to opposite effect [17].

The AdipoR2 was located on the surface of Leydig cells, while AdipoR1 was found in the epithelium of the seminiferous tubules. In spermatozoa there are both types of the adiponectin receptors [17, 148, 149]. The *AdipoR2*$^{-/-}$ mice had the reduced mass and size of testicles, the atrophy of the seminiferous tubules and the impaired spermatogenesis [150]. The expression of AdipoR2 in Leydig cells is controlled by gonadotropins with LH activity, and is almost independent of FSH. The expression of the *AdipoR2* gene in the testes is strongly reduced in hypophysectomized rats, and the treatment of animals with hCG completely restores it [17]. Studying the male rats, it was shown that during puberty with an increase in plasma LH level the expression of AdipoR2 in the testes also increases, which positively correlates with an increase in the adiponectin expression. With regard to the adiponectin signaling in spermatozoa, it is shown that, in addition to adiponectin, both types of adiponectin receptors are expressed in them. The expression of the *Adiponectin*, *AdipoR1* and *AdipoR2* genes in the high-mobility spermatozoa fractions is 3.5, 3.6 and 2.5 times higher in comparison with the low-mobility fraction [149]. The most pronounced correlation was found between the mobility and the expression of the *Adiponectin* and *AdipoR1* genes. These data indicate that AdipoR1 plays an important role in the regulation of spermatogenesis, while AdipoR2 is very important for the T synthesis by Leydig cells.

All of the above indicates that adiponectin positively regulates the T synthesis (**Figure 2**). Indeed, treatment of the MA-10 Leydig cells with adiponectin at the concentrations of 50–5000 ng/mL resulted in an increase in the production of progesterone, a precursor of T, which was associated with cAMP-dependent activation of StAR and cytochrome $P450_{scc}$ [151]. In the earlier studies, it was shown that adiponectin, acting on the testes, suppressed both the basal and hCG-stimulated T production, although the expression of the steroidogenesis enzymes, such as cytochrome $P450_{scc}$ and dehydrogenases 3β-HSD and 17β-HSD3, did not change [17, 148]. The mechanisms of adiponectin action on Leydig cells include the stimulation of PI3K and Akt kinase, which results in the changed expression of Akt-dependent genes, as well as the regulation of ERK1/2, whose activity decreases at low concentrations of adiponectin and increases at its high concentrations [148]. It can be assumed that the dependence of adiponectin effect on ERK1/2 on its concentration, as well as a set of the effector components of MAPK cascade regulated by adiponectin are responsible for the different mode of the regulation of steroidogenesis by this adipokine. The treatment of Leydig cells with adiponectin did not affect the expression of LH receptor, and this indicates the preservation of the sensitivity of these cells to gonadotropins [148].

4. Visfatin

Visfatin produced by the adipose tissue is a multifunctional protein that functions as a signal molecule and as a nicotinamide phosphoribosyltransferase (NAMPT) catalyzing the synthesis of nicotinamide adenine mononucleotide from nicotinamide and 5-phosphoribosyl-1-pyrophosphate [152–154]. In humans, visfatin includes 491 amino acids and forms a functionally active homodimer complex [10, 155, 156]. Paradoxically, the receptor for visfatin has not yet been found. It is known that the main targets of visfatin, as in the case of most other adipokines, are the MAPK and PI3K/Akt pathway, and the activation of Akt kinase occurs 5 min after treatment of cells with visfatin [156–158].

The highest concentration of visfatin is detected in the white adipose tissue. In obesity and DM2, the plasma visfatin level is steadily increased, and the degree of this increase varies greatly, due to both the individual characteristics of patients and the various approaches to measure the visfatin concentration [2, 155]. The visfatin level is also increases in women with a polycystic ovary syndrome, for which obesity and insulin resistance are characteristic [155]. Despite an increase in the plasma level of visfatin, its concentration in the CSF decreases, and this is probably due to the impaired transport of visfatin through the BBB. These data suggest that, as in the case of leptin and insulin, the transport of visfatin into the brain can be receptor-mediated, and decreases in the conditions of visfatin resistance.

The data on the involvement of visfatin in regulation of the reproductive system are mainly related to the female HPG axis, folliculogenesis and steroidogenesis in the ovaries [7]. There is a positive correlation between the visfatin level in follicular fluid and the quantity and quality of the follicles [159]. It is assumed that the effect of visfatin on the ovarian steroidogenesis system can be realized via the mechanisms that lead to an increase in the production of insulin-like growth factor-1 (IGF-1), a stimulator of steroidogenesis [138]. In this case, the effects of visfatin are characterized by species specificity. The introduction of recombinant human visfatin into chicken did not stimulate, but, on the contrary, suppressed the basal and IGF-1-stimulated expression of the *Star* and *Hsd3b1* genes, which led to a decrease in estrogens production by follicular cells [7].

In the case of the male reproductive axis, the targets for visfatin may be all of its components. Information on the central mechanisms of action of visfatin is limited to its effect on the hypothalamic neurons responsible for control of glucose homeostasis [160]. However, the fact that visfatin, like leptin, affects the activity of 3-phosphoinositide pathway, supports its possible participation in the regulation of GnRH-neurons activity. The evidences were obtained in favor of the regulation of LH-expressing pituitary gonadotrophs by visfatin. Firstly, the mRNA for visfatin was detected in gonadotrophs, which indicates its synthesis in them and the role of visfatin in the autocrine and paracrine regulation of the anterior pituitary. Secondly, visfatin stimulates the AMPK activity in the cultured murine gonadotroph-like cells LβT2, resulting in a decrease in LH secretion [161].

The ability of visfatin to influence the testicular functions and the T synthesis is supported by the following data. Visfatin is expressed in Leydig cells, spermatocytes and spermatozoa [19], and its level in the seminal fluid is much higher than in the blood [162]. When exposed to Leydig cells, visfatin increases the T production, and the maximal effect of visfatin is achieved at its concentration of 10^{-6} M [163]. The inhibitor of Raf-1 kinase reduces the stimulating effect of visfatin on steroidogenesis, while the inhibitors of the protein kinases A and C have a little influence on this effect. It is assumed that the effects of visfatin on steroidogenesis may be due to activation of insulin receptors [163], which are widely represented in Leydig cells, especially since previously it has been reported that insulin receptor can interact with visfatin [154, 164]. However, despite the similarity of regulatory effects of insulin and visfatin, in the recent years the ability of visfatin specifically binds to insulin receptor has been questioned [157].

5. Resistin

Resistin is a polypeptide with a molecular mass of 12.5 kDa, which forms a homodimer stabilized by disulfide bonds [138]. Although resistin is mainly secreted by adipocytes of the white and brown adipose tissues and macrophages [165, 166], its expression is also shown in the testes in the Sertoli and Leydig cells, which indicates the participation of resistin in the autocrine and paracrine regulation of testicular cells [16]. The expression of the *Resistin* gene was detected in the different lines of mouse Leydig cells, and it increased with increasing intracellular level of cAMP, which indicates the involvement of cAMP-dependent transcription factors in the regulation of the *Resistin* gene expression [3]. Currently, a specific receptor for resistin is not established, but the most acceptable candidate for this is Toll-like receptor 4 (TLR4) [167]. The functions of receptor proteins for resistin can also be performed by tyrosine kinase-like orphan receptor 1 (ROR1), adenylyl cyclase-associated protein-1 (CAP-1) and δ-decorin. The TLR4 receptor mediates the regulatory effects of resistin on the 3-phosphoinositide and MAPK pathways, AMPK and the transcription factors of the STAT family [3].

The level of resistin in the bloodstream, from which it is able to be transported to the testes, varies greatly depending on the metabolic status, gender and species. Fasting leads to a decrease in the plasma resistin level and the *Resistin* gene expression in the adipose tissue, while food intake increases these indices [9, 16]. In women, the resistin level in the blood is higher than in men [168, 169]. In male rats, the expression of the *Resistin* gene in the adipose tissue exceeds that in female rats [170]. This is believed to be due to the stimulating effect of T and the inhibitory effect of estrogens on adipocytes [171]. There is evidence that resistin is expressed in adenohypophysis cells [172, 173]. In the pituitary of rhesus monkeys and baboons, the ratio of the mRNA for resistin, leptin and adiponectin was 1:13:4 and 1:7:3, respectively [174]. The *Resistin* expression in the pituitary strongly depends on the age and gender, and was higher in males as compared to females and increased at the prepubertal stage [172, 173].

Using the primary culture of pituitary cells of rhesus monkey it was shown that resistin activates a number of signaling pathways, including cAMP-dependent and 3-phosphoinositide cascades regulating the cell survival and secretory activity. Resistin affects the secretion of growth hormone and adrenocorticotropic hormone, although LH secretion remains unchanged. It should be noted, however, that the treatment of pituitary cells with leptin and adiponectin also did not affect LH secretion, which is probably due to the peculiarities of cultured cells used in the experiment [174].

Resistin was found in the brain and CSF, and although its concentration was much lower than in the bloodstream, it can be assumed that resistin affects the activity of hypothalamic neurons controlling GnRH secretion [116, 133]. One of the mechanisms of this may be the influence of resistin on the adiponectin signaling in hypothalamic neurons. A prolonged i.c.v. administration of resistin into rats and mice results in a decrease in the expression of both types of adiponectin receptors, AdipoR1 and AdipoR2, and also reduces the functional activity of APPL-1 protein, thereby weakening the APPL-1-mediated adiponectin signaling. There is reason to believe that this effect of resistin is implemented through the receptor TLR4, since the inhibiting effect of resistin on the adiponectin signaling was not detected in mice lacking TLR4 [175].

The *Resistin* gene is expressed in Leydig cells, and the intratesticular expression of resistin was identified throughout postnatal development with a maximum in adult animals [16]. Resistin is also expressed in Sertoli cells, but its level in them is significantly lower than in Leydig cells. Fasting and i.c.v. administration of leptin lead to a significant decrease in the intratesticular level of resistin, while in diet-induced obesity the expression of resistin in the testes remained unchanged [16]. These data indicate a positive correlation between the levels of resistin in the blood and in the testes. This gives reason to believe that, along with intratesticular synthesis of resistin, the plasma adipokine can be transferred through BTB into the testes, and the receptor TLR4, which are capable of binding to resistin and widely presented in testicular cells may be involved in this process.

6. Conclusion and future perspectives

The regulation of the male gonadal axis by adipokines can be carried out both through the changes in the plasma level and bioavailability of adipokines produced (a systemic regulation) and through the changes in the expression and specific activity of adipokines in the target tissues, the components of the HPG axis, such as the hypothalamus, pituitary and testes (an autonomous regulation). In the case of systemic adipokines regulation, the changes in the plasma level of adipokines that are associated with feeding behavior, physiological conditions, and also with an imbalance of adipokines and a resistance to them in obesity, DM2 and other metabolic disorders directly affect the functional activity of the male HPG axis and T production. Of great importance is the activity of the adipokine-transporting system, which transfers the adipokines through the BBB into the brain, where they regulate the GnRH- and KNDy-neurons involved in GnRH secretion, and also through the BTB into the testes, where they control the steroidogenesis system and the synthesis of T, the main effector hormone of the male HPG axis. In the case of autonomous regulation, the adipokines synthesized in the pituitary and testes function as the autocrine and paracrine factors and to a large extent determine functional activity of the components of the HPG axis. On the one hand, they regulate proliferation and survival of gonadotrophs and testicular cells, primarily Leydig cells, and on the other, affect their ability to produce gonadotropins and steroid hormones. It is important to note that between the systemic and autonomous adipokine-mediated regulation of the male HPG axis there are the complex integrative relationships and interactions that are realized at different levels of this axis. As a consequence, the changes in the pattern and levels of adipokines in the bloodstream can be differently associated with activity of the hypothalamic, pituitary and testicular components of the HPG axis, since in this case it is necessary to take into account the functional state of autonomous adipokine systems. The ratio of different adipokines in the blood and in the tissues, the components of the HPG axis, contributes significantly to the resulting effects of adipokines on the reproductive system, since their effects on the male HPG axis, including the testicular steroidogenesis system, may be synergistic or antagonistic.

The study of the role of adipokines in the regulation of the male HPG axis is of great interest, since it will allow in the future to develop the effective approaches for monitoring functional activity of the male reproductive system and correcting the dysfunctions in this system in metabolic and endocrine disorders, including obesity and DM2. The adipokines and their analogues, as well as regulators and modulators of their signaling cascades in the hypothalamic neurons and testes, can be used as potential drugs to improve the reproductive functions and to normalize the steroidogenesis in men. It is also important how the treatment of men with GnRH analogous, gonadotropins with LH-like activity and androgens will affect the systemic and autonomic regulation of the GPH axis by adipokines. This should be taken into account when developing the approaches to improve metabolic status in obese and diabetic patients and in elderly men with an androgen deficiency using the activators of the HPG axis and androgens. The study of the interaction between the male HPG axis and the adipokine system will allow us to decipher the fundamental mechanisms that determine the relationships between the eating behavior, hunger and satiety, on the one hand, and the sexual behavior and aggression, on the other.

Acknowledgements

This work was supported by the Russian Foundation of Basic Investigations (project No 18-515-45004 IND-a).

Disclosure

Conflicts of interest are absent.

Author details

Alexander O. Shpakov*, Julian R. Ryzhov, Andrey A. Bakhtyukov and Kira V. Derkach

*Address all correspondence to: alex_shpakov@list.ru

Sechenov Institute of Evolutionary Physiology and Biochemistry, Russian Academy of Sciences, St. Petersburg, Russia

References

[1] Roa J, Tena-Sempere M. Connecting metabolism and reproduction: Roles of central energy sensors and key molecular mediators. Molecular and Cellular Endocrinology. 2014;**397**(1-2):4-14. DOI: 10.1016/j.mce.2014.09.027

[2] Dupont J, Pollet-Villard X, Reverchon M, Mellouk N, Levy R. Adipokines in human reproduction. Hormone Molecular Biology and Clinical Investigation. 2015;**24**(1):11-24. DOI: 10.1515/hmbci-2015-0034

[3] Roumaud P, Martin LJ. Roles of leptin, adiponectin and resistin in the transcriptional regulation of steroidogenic genes contributing to decreased Leydig cells function in obesity. Hormone Molecular Biology and Clinical Investigation. 2015;**24**(1):25-45. DOI: 10.1515/hmbci-2015-0046

[4] Mounzih K, Lu R, Chehab FF. Leptin treatment rescues the sterility of genetically obese ob/ob males. Endocrinology. 1997;**138**(3):1190-1193. DOI: 10.1210/endo.138.3.5024

[5] Tena-Sempere M, Barreiro ML. Leptin in male reproduction: The testis paradigm. Molecular and Cellular Endocrinology. 2002;**188**(1-2):9-13. PMID: 11911940

[6] Pinto-Fochi ME, Pytlowanciv EZ, Reame V, Rafacho A, Ribeiro DL, Taboga SR, Góes RM. A high-fat diet fed during different periods of life impairs steroidogenesis of rat Leydig cells. Reproduction. 2016;**152**(6):795-808. DOI: 10.1530/REP-16-0072

[7] Diot M, Reverchon M, Ramé C, Baumard Y, Dupont J. Expression and effect of NAMPT (visfatin) on progesterone secretion in hen granulosa cells. Reproduction. 2015;**150**(1):53-63. DOI: 10.1530/REP-15-0021

[8] Landry D, Cloutier F, Martin L. Implications of leptin in neuroendocrine regulation of male reproduction. Reproductive Biology. 2013;**13**(1):1-14. DOI: 10.1016/j.repbio.2012.12.001

[9] Steppan CM, Bailey ST, Bhat S, Brown EJ, Banerjee RR, Wright CM, Patel HR, Ahima RS. Lazar MA. The Hormone Resistin Links Obesity to Diabetes. 2001;**409**(6818):307-312. DOI: 10.1038/35053000

[10] Stastny J, Bienertova-Vasku J, Vasku A. Visfatin and its role in obesity development. Diabetes & Metabolic Syndrome. 2012;**6**(2):120-124. DOI: 10.1016/j.dsx.2012.08.011

[11] Garcia-Galiano D, Allen SJ, Elias CF. Role of the adipocyte-derived hormone leptin in reproductive control. Hormone Molecular Biology and Clinical Investigation. 2014;**19**(3):141-149. DOI: 10.1515/hmbci-2014-0017

[12] Nagatani S, Guthikonda P, Thompson RC, Tsukamura H, Maeda KI, Foster DL. Evidence for GnRH regulation by leptin: Leptin administration prevents reduced pulsatile LH secretion during fasting. Neuroendocrinology. 1998;**67**(6):370-376. PMID: 9662716

[13] Cheng XB, Wen JP, Yang J, Yang Y, Ning G, Li XY. GnRH secretion is inhibited by adiponectin through activation of AMP-activated protein kinase and extracellular signal-regulated kinase. Endocrine. 2011;**39**(1):6-12. DOI: 10.1007/s12020-010-9375-8

[14] Lu M, Tang Q, Olefsky JM, Mellon PL, Webster NJ. Adiponectin activates adenosine monophosphate-activated protein kinase and decreases luteinizing hormone secretion in LβT2 gonadotropes. Molecular Endocrinology. 2008;**22**(3):760-771. DOI: 10.1210/me.2007-0330

[15] Akhter N, Johnson BW, Crane C, Iruthayanathan M, Zhou YH, Kudo A, Childs GV. Anterior pituitary leptin expression changes in different reproductive states: In vitro stimulation by gonadotropin releasing hormone. The Journal of Histochemistry and Cytochemistry: Official Journal of the Histochemistry Society. 2007;**55**(2):151-166. DOI: 10.1369/jhc.6A7072.2006

[16] Nogueiras R, Barreiro ML, Caminos JE, Gaytán F, Suominen JS, Navarro VM, Casanueva FF, Aguilar E, Toppari J, Diéguez C, Tena-Sempere M. Novel expression of resistin in rat testis: Functional role and regulation by nutritional status and hormonal factors. Journal of Cell Science. 2004;**117**(Pt 15):3247-3257. DOI: 10.1242/jcs.01196

[17] Caminos JE, Nogueiras R, Gaytán F, Pineda R, González CR, Barreiro ML, Castaño JP, Malagón MM, Pinilla L, Toppari J, Diéguez C, Tena-Sempere M. Novel expression and direct effects of adiponectin in the rat testis. Endocrinology. 2008;**149**(7):3390-3402. DOI: 10.1210/en.2007-1582

[18] Rago V, Aquila S, Guido C, Carpino A. Leptin and its receptor are expressed in the testis and in the epididymis of young and adult pigs. Anatomical Record (Hoboken, NJ: 2007). 2009;**292**(5):736-745. DOI: 10.1002/ar.20880

[19] Gurusubramanian G, Roy VK. Expression of visfatin in alloxan-induced diabetic rat testis. Acta Histochemica. 2014;**116**(8):1462-1468. DOI: 10.1016/j.acthis.2014.09.011

[20] Balaskó M, Soós S, Székely M, Pétervári E. Leptin and aging: Review and questions with particular emphasis on its role in the central regulation of energy balance. Journal of Chemical Neuroanatomy. 2014;**61-62**:248-255. DOI: 10.1016/j.jchemneu.2014.08.006

[21] Park HK, Ahima RS. Physiology of leptin: Energy homeostasis, neuroendocrine function and metabolism. Metabolism, Clinical and Experimental. 2015;**64**(1):24-34. DOI: 10.1016/j.metabol.2014.08.004

[22] Paz-Filho G, Mastronardi CA, Licinio J. Leptin treatment: Facts and expectations. Metabolism, Clinical and Experimental. 2015;**64**(1):146-156. DOI: 10.1016/j.metabol.2014.07.014

[23] Munzberg H, Morrison C. Structure, production and signaling of leptin. Metabolism, Clinical and Experimental. 2015;**64**(1):13-23. DOI: 10.1016/j.metabol.2014.09.010

[24] Sáinz N, Barrenetxe J, Moreno-Aliaga MJ, Martínez JA. Leptin resistance and diet-induced obesity: Central and peripheral actions of leptin. Metabolism, Clinical and Experimental. 2015;**64**(1):35-46. DOI: 10.1016/j.metabol.2014.10.015

[25] Zieba DA, Amstalden M, Williams GL. Regulatory roles of leptin in reproduction and metabolism: A comparative review. Domestic Animal Endocrinology. 2005;**29**(1):166-185. DOI: 10.1016/j.domaniend.2005.02.019

[26] Ramos CF, Zamoner A. Thyroid hormone and leptin in the testis. Frontiers in Endocrinology. 2014;**5**:198. DOI: 10.3389/fendo.2014.00198

[27] Mercer JG, Hoggard N, Williams LM, Lawrence CB, Hannah LT, Trayhurn P. Localization of leptin receptor mRNA and the long form splice variant (Ob-Rb) in mouse hypothalamus and adjacent brain regions by in situ hybridization. FEBS Letters. 1996;**387**(2-3):113-116. DOI: 10.1016/0014-5793(96)00473-5

[28] Smith GD, Jackson LM, Foster DL. Leptin regulation of reproduction function and fertility. Theriogenology. 2002;**57**(1):73-86. DOI: https://doi.org/10.1016/S0093-691X(01)00658-6

[29] Hileman S, Pierroz D, Masuzaki H, Bjorbaek C, El-Haschimi K, Banks W, Flier J. Characterization of short isoforms of the leptin receptor in rat cerebral microvessels and of brain uptake of leptin in mouse models of obesity. Endocrinology. 2002;**143**(3):775-783. DOI: 10.1210/endo.143.3.8669

[30] Tu H, Kastin AJ, Hsuchou H, Pan W. Soluble receptor inhibits leptin transport. Journal of Cellular Physiology. 2008;**214**(2):301-305. DOI: 10.1002/jcp.21195

[31] Myers MG, Cowley MA, Münzberg H. Mechanisms of leptin action and leptin resistance. Annual Review of Physiology. 2008;**70**:537-556. DOI: 10.1146/annurev.physiol.70.113006.100707

[32] Shpakov AO. The brain leptin signaling system and its functional state in metabolic syndrome and type 2 diabetes mellitus. Journal of Evolutionary Biochemistry and Physiology. 2016;**52**(3):177-195. DOI: 10.1134/S0022093016030017

[33] Roa J, Garcia-Galiano D, Varela L, Sánchez-Garrido MA, Pineda R, Castellano JM, Ruiz-Pino F, Romero M, Aguilar E, López M, Gaytan F, Diéguez C, Pinilla L, Tena-Sempere M. The mammalian target of rapamycin as novel central regulator of puberty onset via modulation of hypothalamic Kiss1 system. Neuroendocrinology. 2009;**150**(11):5016-5026. DOI: 10.1210/en.2009-0096

[34] Roa J, Aguilar E, Dieguez C, Pinilla L, Tena-Sempere M. New frontiers in kisspeptin/GPR54 physiology as fundamental gatekeepers of reproductive function. Frontiers in Neuroendocrinology. 2008;**29**(1):48-69. DOI: 10.1016/j.yfrne.2007.07.002

[35] Tena-Sempere M. Kisspeptins and the metabolic control of reproduction: Physiologic roles and physiopathological implications. Annales d'Endocrinologie. 2010;**71**(3):201-202. DOI: 10.1016/j.ando.2010.02.018

[36] White CL, Whittington A, Barnes MJ, Wang Z, Bray GA, Morrison CD. HF diets increase hypothalamic PTP1B and induce leptin resistance through both leptin-dependent and -independent mechanisms. American Journal of Physiology. Endocrinology and Metabolism. 2009;**296**(2):E291-E299. DOI: 10.1152/ajpendo.90513.2008

[37] Caprio M, Fabbrini E, Isidori AM, Aversa A, Fabbri A. Leptin in reproduction. Trends in Endocrinology and Metabolism. 2001;**12**(2):65-72. DOI: https://doi.org/10.1016/S1043-2760(00)00352-0

[38] Barash IA, Cheung CC, Weigle DS, Ren H, Kabigting EB, Kuijper JL, Clifton DK, Steiner RA. Leptin is a metabolic signal to the reproductive system. Endocrinology. 1996;**137**(7):3144-3147. DOI: 10.1210/endo.137.7.8770941

[39] Chehab FF, Lim ME, Lu R. Correction of the sterility defect in homozygous obese female mice by treatment with the human recombinant leptin. Nature Genetics. 1996;**12**(3):318-320. DOI: 10.1038/ng0396-318

[40] Strobel A, Issad T, Camoin L, Ozata M, Strosberg AD. A leptin missense mutation associated with hypogonadism and morbid obesity. Nature Genetics. 1998;**18**(3):213-215. DOI: 10.1038/ng0398-213

[41] Farooqi IS. Leptin and the onset of puberty: Insights from rodent and human genetics. Seminars in Reproductive Medicine. 2002;**20**(2):139-144. DOI: 10.1055/s-2002-32505

[42] Hodžić A, Ristanović M, Zorn B, Tulić C, Maver A, Novaković I, Plaseska-Karanfilska D, Peterlin B. Genetic variation in leptin and leptin receptor genes as a risk factor for idiopathic male infertility. Andrology. 2017;**5**(1):70-74. DOI: 10.1111/andr.12295

[43] Khosropour S, Hamidi M, Fattahi A, Khodadadi I, Karami M, Fazilati M, Vaisi-Raygani A, Tavilani H. Leptin and leptin-receptor polymorphisms in fertile and infertile men. Systems Biology in Reproductive Medicine. 2017;**63**(1):7-14. DOI: 10.1080/19396368.2016.1258741

[44] Clément K, Vaisse C, Lahlou N, Cabrol S, Pelloux V, Cassuto D, Dina GM, Chambaz J, Lacorte JM, Basdevant A, Bougnères P, Lebouc Y, Froguel P, Guy-Grand B. A mutation in the human leptin receptor gene causes obesity and pituitary dysfunction. Nature. 1998;**392**(6674):398-401. DOI: 10.1038/32911

[45] Salem H, Rosenfeld T, Altarescu G, Grisaru-Granovsky S, Birk R. Maternal and neonatal leptin and leptin receptor polymorphisms associated with preterm birth. Gene. 2016;**591**(1):209-213. DOI: 10.1016/j.gene.2016.07.014

[46] Yu WH, Kimura M, Walczewska A, Karanth S, McCann SM. Role of leptin in hypothalamic-pituitary function. Proceedings of the National Academy of Sciences of the United States of America. 1997;**94**(3):1023-1028. PMID: 9023376

[47] Amstalden M, Garcia MR, Stanko RL, Nizielski SE, Morrison CD, Keisler DH, Williams GL. Central infusion of recombinant ovine leptin normalizes plasma insulin and stimulates a novel hypersecretion of luteinizing hormone after short-term fasting in mature beef cows. Biology of Reproduction. 2002;**66**(5):1555-1561. PMID: 11967223

[48] Henry BA, Goding JW, Alexander WS, Tilbrook AJ, Canny BJ, Dunshea F, Rao A, Mansell A, Clarke IJ. Central administration of leptin to ovariectomized ewes inhibits food intake without affecting the secretion of hormones from the pituitary gland: Evidence for a dissociation of effects on appetite and neuroendocrine function. Endocrinology. 1999;**140**(3):1175-1182. DOI: 10.1210/endo.140.3.6604

[49] Amstalden M, Zieba DA, Edwards JF, Harms PG, Welsh TH Jr, Stanko RL, Williams GL. Leptin acts at the bovine adenohypophysis to enhance basal and gonadotropin-releasing hormone-mediated release of luteinizing hormone: Differential effects are dependent upon nutritional history. Biology of Reproduction. 2003;**69**(5):1539-1544. DOI: 10.1095/biolreprod.103.018119

[50] Hausman GJ, Barb CR, Lents CA. Leptin and reproductive function. Biochimie. 2012; **94**(10):2075-2081. DOI: 10.1016/j.biochi.2012.02.022

[51] Loram LC, Culp ME, Connolly-Strong EC, Sturgill-Koszycki S. Melanocortin peptides: Potential targets in systemic lupus erythematosus. Inflammation. 2015;**38**(1):260-271. DOI: 10.1007/s10753-014-0029-5

[52] Watanobe H. Leptin directly acts within the hypothalamus to stimulate gonadotropin-releasing hormone secretion in vivo in rats. The Journal of Physiology. 2002;**545**(Pt 1): 255-268. DOI: 10.1113/jphysiol.2002.023895

[53] Roa J, Herbison AE. Direct regulation of GnRH neuron excitability by arcuate nucleus POMC and NPY neuron neuropeptides in female mice. Endocrinology. 2012;**153**(11):5587-5599. DOI: 10.1210/en.2012-1470

[54] Roa J. Role of GnRH neurons and their neuronal afferents as key integrators between food intake regulatory signals and the control of reproduction. International Journal of Endocrinology. 2013;**2013**:518046. DOI: 10.1155/2013/518046

[55] Sandrock M, Schulz A, Merkwitz C, Schöneberg T, Spanel-Borowski K, Ricken A. Reduction in corpora lutea number in obese melanocortin-4-receptor-deficient mice. Reproductive biology and endocrinology: RB&E. 2009;**7**:24. DOI: 10.1186/1477-7827-7-24

[56] Begriche K, Levasseur PR, Zhang J, Rossi J, Skorupa D, Solt LA, Young B, Burris TP, Marks DL, Mynatt RL, Butler AA. Genetic dissection of the functions of the melanocortin-3 receptor, a seven-transmembrane G-protein-coupled receptor, suggests roles for central and peripheral receptors in energy homeostasis. The Journal of Biological Chemistry. 2011;**286**(47):40771-40781. DOI: 10.1074/jbc.M111.278374

[57] Manfredi-Lozano M, Roa J, Ruiz-Pino F, Piet R, Garcia-Galiano D, Pineda R, Zamora A, Leon S, Sanchez-Garrido MA, Romero-Ruiz A, Dieguez C, Vazquez MJ, Herbison AE, Pinilla L, Tena-Sempere M. Defining a novel leptin-melanocortin-kisspeptin pathway

involved in the metabolic control of puberty. Molecular Metabolism. 2016;**5**(10):844-857. DOI: 10.1016/j.molmet.2016.08.003

[58] Ratra DV, Elias CF. Chemical identity of hypothalamic neurons engaged by leptin in reproductive control. Journal of Chemical Neuroanatomy. 2014;**61-62**:233-238. DOI: 10.1016/j.jchemneu.2014.05.005

[59] Egan OK, Inglis MA, Anderson GM. Leptin signaling in AgRP neurons modulates puberty onset and adult fertility in mice. The Journal of Neuroscience: The Official Journal of the Society for Neuroscience. 2017;**37**(14):3875-3886. DOI: 10.1523/JNEUROSCI.3138-16.2017

[60] Gamba M, Pralong FP. Control of GnRH neuronal activity by metabolic factors: The role of leptin and insulin. Molecular and Cellular Endocrinology. 2006;**254-255**:133-139. DOI: 10.1016/j.mce.2006.04.023

[61] Pierroz DD, Gruaz NM, d'Alièves V, Aubert ML. Chronic administration of neuropeptide Y into the lateral ventricle starting at 30 days of life delays sexual maturation in the female rat. Neuroendocrinology. 1995;**61**(3):293-300. PMID: 7898634

[62] Gonzales C, Voirol MJ, Giacomini M, Gaillard RC, Pedrazzini T, Pralong FP. The neuropeptide Y Y1 receptor mediates NPY-induced inhibition of the onadotrope axis under poor metabolic conditions. The FASEB Journal. 2004;**18**(1):137-139. DOI: 10.1096/fj.03-0189fje

[63] Crown A, Clifton DC, Steiner RA. Neuropeptide signaling in the integration of metabolism andreproduction. Neuroendocrinology. 2007;**86**(3):175-182. DOI: 10.1159/000109095

[64] Muroi Y, Ishii T. A novel neuropeptide Y neuronal pathway linking energy state and reproductive behavior. Neuropeptides. 2016;**59**:1-8. DOI: 10.1016/j.npep.2016.09.002

[65] Shpakov AO, Derkach KV, Berstein LM. Brain signaling systems in the type 2 diabetes and metabolic syndrome: Promising target to treat and prevent these diseases. Future Science OA. 2015;**1**(3):FSO25. DOI: 10.4155/fso.15.23

[66] Mathew H, Castracane VD, Mantzoros C. Adipose tissue and reproductive health. Metabolism. 2017; pii: S0026-0495(17)30309-8. DOI: 10.1016/j.metabol.2017.11.006

[67] Jin L, Zhang S, Burguera BG, Couce ME, Osamura RY, Kulig E, Lloyd RV. Leptin and leptin receptor expression in rat and mouse pituitary cells. Endocrinology. 2000;**141**(1):333-339. DOI: 10.1210/endo.141.1.7260

[68] Kaminski T, Smolinska N, Gajewska A, Siawrys G, Okrasa S, Kochman K, Przala J. Leptin and long form of leptin receptor genes expression in the hypothalamus and pituitary during the luteal phase and early pregnancy in pigs. Journal of Physiology and Pharmacology: An Official Journal of the Polish Physiological Society. 2006;**57**(1):95-108. PMID: 16601318

[69] Akhter N, Crane C, Childs GV. Pituitary leptin – a paracrine regulator of gonadotropes: A review. The Open Neuroendocrinology Journal. 2011;**4**:25-42

[70] Odle AK, Haney A, Allensworth-James M, Akhter N, Childs GV. Adipocyte versus pituitary leptin in the regulation of pituitary hormones: Somatotropes develop normally in the absence of circulating leptin. Endocrinology. 2014;**155**(11):4316-4328. DOI: 10.1210/en.2014-1172

[71] Sone M, Osamura RY. Leptin and the pituitary. Pituitary. 2001;**4**(1-2):15-23. PMID: 11824504

[72] McDuffie IA, Akhter N, Childs GV. Regulation of leptin mRNA and protein expression in pituitary somatotropes. The Journal of Histochemistry and Cytochemistry: Official Journal of the Histochemistry Society. 2004;**52**(2):263-273. DOI: 10.1177/002215540405200214

[73] Odle AK, Beneš H, Melgar Castillo A, Akhter N, Syed M, Haney A, Allensworth-James M, Hardy L, Winter B, Manoharan R, Syed R, MacNicol MC, MacNicol AM, Childs GV. Association of GnRHR mRNA with the stem cell determinant musashi: A mechanism for leptin-mediated modulation of GnRHR expression. Endocrinology. 2018;**159**(2):883-894. DOI: 10.1210/en.2017-00586

[74] Iqbal J, Pompolo S, Considine RV, Clarke IJ. Localization of leptin receptor-like immunoreactivity in the corticotropes, somatotropes, and gonadotropes in the ovine anterior pituitary. Endocrinology. 2000;**141**(4):1515-1520. DOI: 10.1210/endo.141.4.7433

[75] Banks WA, McLay RN, Kastin AJ, Sarmiento U, Scully S. Passage of leptin across the blood-testis barrier. The American Journal of Physiology. 1999;**276**(Pt 1):E1099-E1104

[76] Herrid M, O'Shea T, McFarlane JR. Ontogeny of leptin and its receptor expression in mouse testis during the postnatal period. Molecular Reproduction and Development. 2008;**75**(5):874-880. DOI: 10.1002/mrd.20796

[77] Caprio M, Fabbrini E, Ricci G, Basciani S, Gnessi L, Arizzi M, Carta AR, De Martino MU, Isidori AM, Frajese GV, Fabbri A. Ontogenesis of leptin receptor in rat Leydig cells. Biology of Reproduction 2003;**68**(4):1199-1207. DOI: 10.1095/biolreprod.102.007831

[78] Ishikawa T, Fujioka H, Ishimura T, Takenaka A, Fujisawa M. Expression of leptin and leptin receptor in the testis of fertile and infertile patients. Andrologia. 2007;**39**(1):22-27. DOI: 10.1111/j.1439-0272.2006.00754.x

[79] Müller L, Kowalewski MP, Reichler IM, Kollár E, Balogh O. Different expression of leptin and IGF1 in the adult and prepubertal testis in dogs. Reproduction in domestic animals =. Zuchthygiene. 2017;**52**(2):187-192. DOI: 10.1111/rda.12896

[80] Caprio M, Isidori AM, Carta AR, Moretti C, Dufau ML, Fabbri A. Expression of functional leptin receptors in rodent Leydig cells. Endocrinology. 1999;**140**(11):4939-4947. DOI: 10.1210/endo.140.11.7088

[81] Schanton M, Maymó JL, Pérez-Pérez A, Sánchez-Margalet V, Varone CL. Involvement of leptin in the molecular physiology of the placenta. Reproduction. 2018;**155**(1):R1-R2. DOI: 10.1530/REP-17-0512

[82] Han YH, Cao X, Lin B, Lin F, Kolluri SK, Stebbins J, Reed JC, Dawson MI, Zhang XK. Regulation of Nur77 nuclear export by c-Jun N-terminal kinase and Akt. Oncogene. 2006;**25**(21):2974-2986. DOI: 10.1038/sj.onc.1209358

[83] Liu B, Wu JF, Zhan YY, Chen HZ, Zhang XY, Wu Q. Regulation of the orphan receptor TR3 nuclear functions by c-Jun N terminal kinase phosphorylation. Endocrinology. 2007;**148**(1):34-44. DOI: 10.1210/en.2006-0800

[84] Manna PR, Dyson MT, Stocco DM. Regulation of the steroidogenic acute regulatory protein gene expression: Present and future perspectives. Molecular Human Reproduction. 2009;**15**(6):321-333. DOI: 10.1093/molehr/gap025

[85] Caron KM, Soo SC, Wetsel WC, Stocco DM, Clark BJ, Parker KL. Targeted disruption of the mouse gene encoding steroidogenic acute regulatory protein provides insights into congenital lipoid adrenal hyperplasia. Proceedings of the National Academy of Sciences of the United States of America. 1997;**94**(21):11540-11545. PMID: 9326645

[86] Chau YM, Crawford PA, Woodson KG, Polish JA, Olson LM, Sadovsky Y. Role of steroidogenic-factor 1 in basal and 3′,5′-cyclic adenosine monophosphate-mediated regulation of cytochrome P450 side-chain cleavage enzyme in the mouse. Biology of Reproduction. 1997;**57**(4):765-771. PMID: 9314578

[87] Leers-Sucheta S, Morohashi K, Mason JI, Melner MH. Synergistic activation of the human type II 3beta-hydroxysteroid dehydrogenase/delta5-delta4 isomerase promoter by the transcription factor steroidogenic factor-1/adrenal 4-binding protein and phorbol ester. The Journal of Biological Chemistry. 1997;**272**(12):7960-7967. DOI: 10.1074/jbc.272.12.7960

[88] Whitby RJ, Stec J, Blind RD, Dixon S, Leesnitzer LM, Orband-Miller LA, Williams SP, Willson TM, Xu R, Zuercher WJ, Cai F, Ingraham HA. Small molecule agonists of the orphan nuclearreceptors steroidogenic factor-1 (SF-1, NR5A1) and liver receptor homologue-1 (LRH-1, NR5A2). Journal of Medicinal Chemistry. 2011;**54**(7):2266-2281. DOI: 10.1021/jm1014296

[89] Bjørbaek C, Buchholz RM, Davis SM, Bates SH, Pierroz DD, Gu H, Neel BG, Myers MG Jr, Flier JS. Divergent roles of SHP-2 in ERK activation by leptin receptors. The Journal of Biological Chemistry. 2001;**276**(7):4747-4755. DOI: 10.1074/jbc.M007439200

[90] Li Y, Xu S, Mihaylova MM, Zheng B, Hou X, Jiang B, Park O, Luo Z, Lefai E, Shyy JY, Gao B, Wierzbicki M, Verbeuren TJ, Shaw RJ, Cohen RA, Zang M. AMPK phosphorylates and inhibits SREBP activity to attenuate hepatic steatosis and atherosclerosis in diet-induced insulin-resistant mice. Cell Metabolsim. 2011;**13**(4):376-388. DOI: 10.1016/j.cmet.2011.03.009

[91] Shea-Eaton WK, Trinidad MJ, Lopez D, Nackley A, McLean MP. Sterol regulatory element binding protein-1a regulation of the steroidogenic acute regulatory protein gene. Endocrinology. 2001;**142**(4):1525-1533. DOI: 10.1210/endo.142.4.8075

[92] Christenson LK, Osborne TF, McAllister JM, Strauss JF 3rd. Conditional response of the human steroidogenic acute regulatory protein gene promoter to sterol regulatory element binding protein-1a. Endocrinology. 2001;**142**(1):28-36. DOI: 10.1210/endo.142.1.7867

[93] Condorelli RA, Calogero AE, Vicari E, Mongioi′ L, Favilla V, Morgia G, Cimino S, Russo G, La Vignera S. The gonadal function in obese adolescents: Review. Journal of Endocrinological Investigation. 2014;**37**(12):1133-1142. DOI: 10.1007/s40618-014-0107-4

[94] Roubos EW, Dahmen M, Kozicz T, Xu L. Leptin and the hypothalamo-pituitary-adrenal stress axis. General and Comparative Endocrinology. 2012;**177**(1):28-36. DOI: 10.1016/j.ygcen.2012.01.009

[95] Cheung KK, Luk AO, So WY, Ma RC, Kong AP, Chow FC, Chan JC. Testosterone level in men with type 2 diabetes mellitus and related metabolic effects: A review of current evidence. Journal of Diabetes Investigation. 2015;**6**(2):112-123. DOI: 10.1111/jdi.12288

[96] Kelly DM, Jones TH. Testosterone and obesity. Obesity Reviews: An Official Journal of the International Association for the Study of Obesity. 2015;**16**(7):581-606. DOI: 10.1111/obr.12282

[97] Taylor SR, Meadowcraft LM, Williamson B. Prevalence, Pathophysiology, and management of androgen deficiency in men with metabolic syndrome, type 2 diabetes mellitus, or both. Pharmacotherapy. 2015;**35**(8):780-792. DOI: 10.1002/phar.1623

[98] Williams G. Aromatase up-regulation, insulin and raised intracellular oestrogens in men, induce adiposity, metabolic syndrome and prostate disease, via aberrant ER-α and GPER signalling. Molecular and Cellular Endocrinology. 2012;**351**(2):269-278. DOI: 10.1016/j.mce.2011.12.017

[99] Holmboe SA, Jensen TK, Linneberg A, Scheike T, Thuesen BH, Skakkebaek NE, Juul A, Andersson AM. Low testosterone: A risk marker rather than a risk factor for type 2 diabetes. The Journal of Clinical Endocrinology and Metabolism. 2016;**101**(8):3180-3190. DOI: 10.1210/jc.2016-1778

[100] Hu J, Zhang A, Yang S, Wang Y, Goswami R, Zhou H, Zhang Y, Wang Z, Li R, Cheng Q, Zhen Q, Li Q. Combined effects of sex hormone-binding globulin and sex hormones on risk of incident type 2 diabetes. Journal of Diabetes. 2016;**8**(4):508-515. DOI: 10.1111/1753-0407.12322

[101] Vihma V, Naukkarinen J, Turpeinen U, Hämäläinen E, Kaprio J, Rissanen A, Heinonen S, Hakkarainen A, Lundbom J, Lundbom N, Mikkola TS, Tikkanen MJ, Pietiläinen KH. Metabolism of sex steroids is influenced by acquired adiposity: A study of young adult male monozygotic twin pairs. The Journal of Steroid Biochemistry and Molecular Biology. 2017;**172**:98-105. DOI: 10.1016/j.jsbmb.2017.06.007

[102] Cunningham GR. Testosterone and metabolic syndrome. Asian Journal of Andrology. 2015;**17**(2):192-196. DOI: 10.4103/1008-682X.148068

[103] Banks WA, Farrell CL. Impaired transport of leptin across the blood-brain barrier in obesity is acquired and reversible. American Journal of Physiology. Endocrinology and Metabolism. 2003;**285**(1):E10-E15. DOI: 10.1152/ajpendo.00468.2002

[104] Romanova IV, Derkach KV, Mikhrina AL, Sukhov IB, Mikhailova EV, Shpakov AO. The leptin, dopamine and serotonin receptors in hypothalamic POMC-neurons in normal and obese rodents. Neurochemical Research. DOI: 10.1007/s11064-018-2485-z

[105] Wagner IV, Klöting N, Atanassova N, Savchuk I, Spröte C, Kiess W, Söder O, Svechnikov K. Prepubertal onset of obesity negatively impacts on testicular steroidogenesis in rats. Molecular and Cellular Endocrinology. 2016;**437**:154-162. DOI: 10.1016/j.mce.2016.08.027

[106] Nelson VL, Negrón AL, Reid I, Thomas JA, Yang L, Lin RZ, Acosta-Martínez M. Loss of PI3K p110α in the adipose tissue results in infertility and delayed puberty onset in male mice. BioMed Research International. 2017;**2017**:3756089. DOI: 10.1155/2017/3756089

[107] Eddy EM, Washburn TF, Bunch DO, Goulding EH, Gladen BC, Lubahn DB, Korach KS. Targeted disruption of the estrogen receptor gene inmale mice causes alteration of spermatogenesis and infertility. Endocrinology. 1996;**137**(11):4796-4805. DOI: 10.1210/endo.137.11.8895349

[108] McDevitt MA, Glidewell-Kenney C, Weiss J, Chambon P, Jameson JL, Levine JE. Estrogen response element-independent estrogen receptor (ER)-α signaling does not rescue sexual behavior but restores normal testosterone secretion in male ERα knockout mice. Endocrinology. 2007;**148**(11):5288-5294. DOI: 10.1210/en.2007-0673

[109] Budak E, Fernández Sánchez M, Bellver J, Cerveró A, Simón C, Pellicer A. Interactions of the hormones leptin, ghrelin, adiponectin, resistin, and PYY3-36 with the reproductive system. Fertility and Sterility. 2006;**85**(6):1563-1581. DOI: 10.1016/j.fertnstert.2005.09.065

[110] Stern JH, Rutkowski JM, Scherer PE. Adiponectin, leptin, and fatty acids in the maintenance of metabolic homeostasis through adipose tissue crosstalk. Cell Metabolism. 2016;**23**(5):770-784. DOI: 10.1016/j.cmet.2016.04.011

[111] Kadowaki T, Yamauchi T. Adiponectin and adiponectin receptors. Endocrine Reviews. 2005;**26**(3):439-451. DOI: 10.1210/er.2005-0005

[112] Nishizawa H, Shimomura I, Kishida K, Maeda N, Kuriyama H, Nagaretani H, Matsuda M, Kondo H, Furuyama N, Kihara S, Nakamura T, Tochino Y, Funahashi T, Matsuzawa Y. Androgens decrease plasma adiponectin, an insulin-sensitizing adipocyte-derived protein. Diabetes. 2002;**51**(9):2734-2741. DOI: https://doi.org/10.2337/diabetes.51.9.2734

[113] Wilkinson M, Brown R, Imran SA, Ur E. Adipokine gene expression in brain and pituitary gland. Neuroendocrinology. 2007;**86**(3):191-209. DOI: 10.1159/000108635

[114] Hu E, Liang P, Spiegelman BM. AdipoQ is a novel adipose-specific gene dysregulated in obesity. The Journal of Biological Chemistry. 1996;**271**(18):10697-10703. DOI: 10.1074/jbc.271.18.10697

[115] Wang Y, Lam KS, Yau MH, Xu A. Post-translational modifications of adiponectin: Mechanisms and functional implications. The Biochemical Journal. 2008;**409**(3):623-633. DOI: 10.1042/BJ20071492

[116] Rak A, Mellouk N, Froment P, Dupont J. Adiponectin and resistin: Potential metabolic signals affecting hypothalamo-pituitary gonadal axis in females and males of different species. Reproduction. 2017;**153**(6):R215-R226. DOI: 10.1530/REP-17-0002

[117] Shapiro L, Scherer PE. The crystal structure of a complement-1q family protein suggests an evolutionary link to tumor necrosis factor. Current Biology. 1998;**8**(6):335-340. DOI: https://doi.org/10.1016/S0960-9822(98)70133-2

[118] Wang Y, Lu G, Wong WP, Vliegenthart JF, Gerwig GJ, Lam KS, Cooper GJ, Xu A. Proteomic and functional characterization of endogenous adiponectin purified from fetal bovine serum. Proteomics. 2004;**4**(12):3933-3942. DOI: 10.1002/pmic.200400826

[119] Richards AA, Stephens T, Charlton HK, Jones A, Macdonald GA, Prins JB, Whitehead JP. Adiponectin multimerization is dependent on conserved lysines in the collagenous domain: Evidence for regulation of multimerization by alterations in posttranslational modifications. Molecular Endocrinology. 2006;**20**(7):1673-1687. DOI: 10.1210/me.2005-0390

[120] Tsao TS, Tomas E, Murrey HE, Hug C, Lee DH, Ruderman NB, Heuser JE, Lodish HF. Role of disulfide bonds in Acrp30/adiponectin structure and signaling specificity. Different oligomers activate different signal transduction pathways. The Journal of Biological Chemistry. 2003;**278**(50):50810-50817. DOI: 10.1074/jbc.M309469200

[121] Fruebis J, Tsao TS, Javorschi S, Ebbets-Reed D, Erickson MR, Yen FT, Bihain BE, Lodish HF. Proteolytic cleavage product of 30-kDa adipocyte complement-related protein increases fatty acid oxidation in muscle and causes weight loss in mice. Proceedings of the National Academy of Sciences of the United States of America. 2001;**98**(4):2005-2010. DOI: 10.1073/pnas.041591798

[122] Waki H, Yamauchi T, Kamon J, Kita S, Ito Y, Hada Y, Uchida S, Tsuchida A, Takekawa S, Kadowaki T. Generation of globular fragment of adiponectin by leukocyte elastase secreted by monocytic cell line THP-1. Endocrinology. 2005;**146**(2):790-796. DOI: 10.1210/en.2004-1096

[123] Martin LJ. Implications of adiponectin in linking metabolism to testicular function. Endocrine. 2014;**46**(1):16-28. DOI: 10.1007/s12020-013-0102-0

[124] Simpson F, Whitehead JP. Adiponectin: It's all about the modifications. The International Journal of Biochemistry & Cell Biology. 2010;**42**(6):785-788. DOI: 10.1016/j.biocel.2009.12.021

[125] Yamauchi T, Iwabu M, Okada-Iwabu M, Kadowaki T. Adiponectin receptors: A review of their structure, function and how they work. Best Practice & Research. Clinical Endocrinology & Metabolism. 2014;**28**(1):15-23. DOI: 10.1016/j.beem.2013.09.003

[126] Yamauchi T, Kamon J, Ito Y, Tsuchida A, Yokomizo T, Kita S, Sugiyama T, Miyagishi M, Hara K, Tsunoda M, Murakami K, Ohteki T, Uchida S, Takekawa S, Waki H, Tsuno NH, Shibata Y, Terauchi Y, Froguel P, Tobe K, Koyasu S, Taira K, Kitamura T, Shimizu T, Nagai R, Kadowaki T. Cloning of adiponectin receptors that mediate antidiabetic metabolic effects. Nature. 2003;**423**(6941):762-769. DOI: 10.1038/nature01705

[127] Yamauchi T, Nio Y, Maki T, Kobayashi M, Takazawa T, Iwabu M, Okada-Iwabu M, Kawamoto S, Kubota N, Kubota T, Ito Y, Kamon J, Tsuchida A, Kumagai K, Kozono H, Hada Y, Ogata H, Tokuyama K, Tsunoda M, Ide T, Murakami K, Awazawa M, Takamoto I, Froguel P, Hara K, Tobe K, Nagai R, Ueki K, Kadowaki T. Targeted disruption of AdipoR1 and AdipoR2 causes abrogation of adiponectin binding and metabolic actions. Nature Medicine. 2007;**13**(3):332-339. DOI: 10.1038/nm1557

[128] Wang C, Xin X, Xiang R, Ramos FJ, Liu M, Lee HJ, Chen H, Mao X, Kikani CK, Liu F, Dong LQ. Yin-Yang regulation of adiponectin signaling by APPL isoforms in muscle cells. The Journal of Biological Chemistry. 2009;**284**(46):31608-31615. DOI: 10.1074/jbc.M109.010355

[129] Liu Z, Xiao T, Peng X, Li G, Hu F. APPLs: More than just adiponectin receptor binding proteins. Cellular Signalling. 2017;**32**:76-84. DOI: 10.1016/j.cellsig.2017.01.018

[130] Combs TP, Marliss EB. Adiponectin signaling in the liver. Reviews in Endocrine & Metabolic Disorders. 2014;**15**(2):137-147. DOI: 10.1007/s11154-013-9280-6

[131] Spranger J, Verma S, Göhring I, Bobbert T, Seifert J, Sindler AL, Pfeiffer A, Hileman SM, Tschöp M, Banks WA. Adiponectin does not cross the blood-brain barrier but modifies cytokine expression of brain endothelial cells. Diabetes. 2006;**55**(1):141-147. DOI: https://doi.org/10.2337/diabetes.55.01.06.db05-1077

[132] Kubota N, Yano W, Kubota T, Yamauchi T, Itoh S, Kumagai H, Kozono H, Takamoto I, Okamoto S, Shiuchi T, Suzuki R, Satoh H, Tsuchida A, Moroi M, Sugi K, Noda T, Ebinuma H, Ueta Y, Kondo T, Araki E, Ezaki O, Nagai R, Tobe K, Terauchi Y, Ueki K, Minokoshi Y, Kadowaki T. Adiponectin stimulates AMP-activated protein kinase in the hypothalamus and increases food intake. Cell Metabolism. 2007;**6**(1):55-68. DOI: 10.1016/j.cmet.2007.06.003

[133] Kos K, Harte AL, da Silva NF, Tonchev A, Chaldakov G, James S, Snead DR, Hoggart B, O'Hare JP, McTernan PG, Kumar S. Adiponectin and resistin in human cerebrospinal fluid and expression of adiponectin receptors in the human hypothalamus. The Journal of Clinical Endocrinology and Metabolism 2007;**92**(3):1129-1136. DOI: 10.1210/jc.2006-1841

[134] Kusminski CM, McTernan PG, Schraw T, Kos K, O'Hare JP, Ahima R, Kumar S, Scherer PE. Adiponectin complexes in human cerebrospinal fluid: Distinct complex distribution from serum. Diabetologia. 2007;**50**(3):634-642. DOI: 10.1007/s00125-006-0577-9

[135] Neumeier M, Weigert J, Buettner R, Wanninger J, Schäffler A, Müller AM, Killian S, Sauerbruch S, Schlachetzki F, Steinbrecher A, Aslanidis C, Schölmerich J, Buechler C. Detection of adiponectin in cerebrospinal fluid in humans. American Journal of Physiology. Endocrinology and Metabolism. 2007;**293**(4):E965-E969. DOI: 10.1152/ajpendo.00119.2007

[136] Staiger H, Tschritter O, Machann J, Thamer C, Fritsche A, Maerker E, Schick F, Häring HU, Stumvoll M. Relationship of serum adiponectin and leptin concentrations with body fat distribution in humans. Obesity Research. 2003;**11**(3):368-372. DOI: 10.1038/oby.2003.48

[137] Böttner A, Kratzsch J, Müller G, Kapellen TM, Blüher S, Keller E, Blüher M, Kiess W. Gender differences of adiponectin levels develop during the progression of puberty and are related to serum androgen levels. The Journal of Clinical Endocrinology and Metabolism. 2004;**89**(8):4053-4061. DOI: 10.1210/jc.2004-0303

[138] Reverchon M, Maillard V, Froment P, Ramé C, Dupont J. Adiponectin and resistin: A role in the reproductive functions? Médecine Sciences: M/S. 2013;**29**(4):417-424. DOI: 10.1051/medsci/2013294016

[139] Wen JP, Lv WS, Yang J, Nie AF, Cheng XB, Yang Y, Ge Y, Li XY, Ning G. Globular adiponectin inhibits GnRH secretion from GT1-7 hypothalamic GnRH neurons by induction of hyperpolarization of membrane potential. Biochemical and Biophysical Research Communications. 2008;**371**(4):756-761. DOI: 10.1016/j.bbrc.2008.04.146

[140] Wen JP, Liu C, Bi WK, Hu YT, Chen Q, Huang H, Liang JX, Li LT, Lin LX, Chen G. Adiponectin inhibits KISS1 gene transcription through AMPK and specificity protein-1 in the hypothalamic GT1-7 neurons. The Journal of Endocrinology. 2012; **214**(2):177-189. DOI: 10.1530/JOE-12-0054

[141] Chu S, Ferro TJ. Sp1: Regulation of gene expression by phosphorylation. Gene. 2005; **348**:1-11. DOI: 10.1016/j.gene.2005.01.013

[142] Psilopanagioti A, Papadaki H, Kranioti EF, Alexandrides TK, Varakis JN. Expression of adiponectin and adiponectin receptors in human pituitary gland and brain. Neuroendocrinology. 2009;**89**(1):38-47. DOI: 10.1159/000151396

[143] Kiezun M, Smolinska N, Maleszka A, Dobrzyn K, Szeszko K, Kaminski T. Adiponectin expression in the porcine pituitary during the estrous cycle and its effect on LH and FSH secretion. American journal of physiology. Endocrinology and Metabolism. 2014;**307**(11):1038-1046. DOI: 10.1152/ajpendo.00299.2014

[144] Rodriguez-Pacheco F, Martinez-Fuentes AJ, Tovar S, Pinilla L, Tena-Sempere M, Dieguez C, Castaño JP, Malagon MM. Regulation of pituitary cell function by adiponectin. Endocrinology. 2007;**148**(1):401-410. DOI: 10.1210/en.2006-1019

[145] Thomas S, Kratzsch D, Schaab M, Scholz M, Grunewald S, Thiery J, Paasch U, Kratzsch J. Seminal plasma adipokine levels are correlated with functional characteristics of spermatozoa. Fertility and Sterility. 2013;**99**(5):1256-1263. DOI: 10.1016/j.fertnstert.2012.12.022

[146] Heinz JF, Singh SP, Janowitz U, Hoelker M, Tesfaye D, Schellander K, Sauerwein H. Characterization of adiponectin concentrations and molecular weight forms in serum, seminal plasma, and ovarian follicular fluid from cattle. Theriogenology. 2015;**83**(3):326-333. DOI: 10.1016/j.theriogenology.2014.06.030

[147] Bai J, Liu Y, Niu GF, Bai LX, Xu XY, Zhang GZ, Wang LX. Relationship between adiponectin and testosterone in patients with type 2 diabetes. Biochemia Medica 2011;21(1):65-70. DOI: http://dx.doi.org/10.11613/BM.2011.013

[148] Pfaehler A, Nanjappa MK, Coleman ES, Mansour M, Wanders D, Plaisance EP, Judd RL, Akingbemi BT. Regulation of adiponectin secretion by soy isoflavones has implication for endocrine function of the testis. Toxicology Letters. 2012;**209**(1):78-85. DOI: 10.1016/j.toxlet.2011.11.027

[149] Kadivar A, Heidari Khoei H, Hassanpour H, Golestanfar A, Ghanaei H. Correlation of adiponectin mRNA abundance and its receptors with quantitative parameters of sperm motility in rams. International Journal of Fertility & Sterility. 2016;**10**(1):127-135. DOI: 10.22074/ijfs.2016.4778

[150] Bjursell M, Ahnmark A, Bohlooly-Y M, William-Olsson L, Rhedin M, Peng XR, Ploj K, Gerdin AK, Arnerup G, Elmgren A, Berg AL, Oscarsson J, Lindén D. Opposing effects of adiponectin receptors 1 and 2 on energy metabolism. Diabetes. 2007;**56**(3):583-593. DOI: 10.2337/db06-1432

[151] Landry D, Paré A, Jean S, Martin LJ. Adiponectin influences progesterone production from MA-10 Leydig cells in a dose-dependent manner. Endocrine. 2015;**48**(3):957-967. DOI: 10.1007/s12020-014-0456-y

[152] Fukuhara A, Matsuda M, Nishizawa M, Segawa K, Tanaka M, Kishimoto K, Matsuki Y, Murakami M, Ichisaka T, Murakami H, Watanabe E, Takagi T, Akiyoshi M, Ohtsubo T, Kihara S, Yamashita S, Makishima M, Funahashi T, Yamanaka S, Hiramatsu R, Matsuzawa Y, Shimomura I. Visfatin: A protein secreted by visceral fat that mimics the effects of insulin. Science. 2005;**307**(5708):426-430. DOI: 10.1126/science.1097243

[153] Chang YH, Chang DM, Lin KC, Shin SJ, Lee YJ. Visfatin in overweight/obesity, type 2 diabetes mellitus, insulin resistance, metabolic syndrome and cardiovascular diseases: A meta-analysis and systemic review. Diabetes/Metabolism Research and Reviews. 2011;**27**(6):515-527. DOI: 10.1002/dmrr.1201

[154] Dahl TB, Holm S, Aukrust P, Halvorsen B. Visfatin/NAMPT: A multifaceted molecule with diverse roles in physiology and pathophysiology. Annual Review of Nutrition. 2012;**32**:229-243. DOI: 10.1146/annurev-nutr-071811-150746

[155] Adeghate E. Visfatin: Structure, function and relation to diabetes mellitus and other dysfunctions. Current Medicinal Chemistry. 2008;**15**(18):1851-1862. DOI: 10.2174/092986708785133004

[156] Sun Z, Lei H, Zhang Z. Pre-b cell colony enhancing factor (PBEF), a cytokine with multiple physiological functions. Cytokine & Growth Factor Reviews. 2013;**24**(5):433-442. DOI: 10.1016/j.cytogfr.2013.05.006

[157] Revollo JR, Körner A, Mills KF, Satoh A, Wang T, Garten A, Dasgupta B, Sasaki Y, Wolberger C, Townsend RR, Milbrandt J, Kiess W, Imai S. Nampt/PBEF/Visfatin regulates insulin secretion in β cells as a systemic NAD biosynthetic enzyme. Cell Metabolism. 2007;**6**(5):363-375. DOI: 10.1016/j.cmet.2007.09.003

[158] Song HK, Lee MH, Kim BK, Park YG, Ko GJ, Kang YS, Han JY, Han SY, Han KH, Kim HK, Cha DR. Visfatin: A new player in mesangial cell physiology anddiabetic nephropathy. American Journal of Physiology. Renal Physiology. 2008;**295**(5):F1485-F1494. DOI: 10.1152/ajprenal.90231.2008

[159] Shen CJ, Tsai EM, Lee JN, Chen YL, Lee CH, Chan TF. The concentrations of visfatin in the follicular fluids of women undergoing controlled ovarian stimulation are correlated to the number of oocytes retrieved. Fertility and Sterility. 2010;**93**(6):1844-1850. DOI: 10.1016/j.fertnstert.2008.12.090

[160] Kim DS, Kang S, Moon NR, Park S. Central visfatin potentiates glucose-stimulated insulin secretion and β-cell mass without increasing serum visfatin levels in diabetic rats. Cytokine. 2014;**65**(2):159-166. DOI: 10.1016/j.cyto.2013.11.008

[161] Maillard V, Elis S, Desmarchais A, Hivelin C, Lardic L, Lomet D, Uzbekova S, Monget P, Dupont J. Visfatin and resistin in gonadotroph cells: Expression, regulation of LH secretion and signalling pathways. Reproduction, Fertility, and Development. 2017;**29**(12):2479-2495. DOI: 10.1071/RD16301

[162] Jeremy M, Gurusubramanian G, Roy VK. Localization pattern of visfatin (NAMPT) in d-galactose induced aged rat testis. Annals of Anatomy = Anatomischer Anzeiger: Official Organ of the Anatomische Gesellschaft. 2017;**211**:46-54. DOI: 10.1016/j.aanat.2017.01.009

[163] Hameed W, Yousaf I, Latif R, Aslam M. Effect of visfatin on testicular steroidogenesis in purified Leydig cells. Journal of Ayub Medical College, Abbottabad: JAMC. 2012;**24**(3-4):62-64. PMID: 24669612

[164] Varma V, Yao-Borengasser A, Rasouli N, Bodles AM, Phanavanh B, Lee MJ, Starks T, Kern LM, Spencer HJ 3rd, McGehee RE Jr, Fried SK, Kern PA. Human visfatin expression: Relationship to insulin sensitivity, intramyocellular lipids, and inflammation. The Journal of Clinical Endocrinology and Metabolism. 2007;**92**(2):666-672. DOI: 10.1210/jc.2006-1303

[165] Kaser S, Kaser A, Sandhofer A, Ebenbichler CF, Tilg H, Patsch JR. Resistin messenger-RNA expression is increased by proinflammatory cytokines in vitro. Biochemical and Biophysical Research Communications. 2003;**309**(2):286-290. DOI: https://doi.org/10.1016/j.bbrc.2003.07.003

[166] Patel L, Buckels AC, Kinghorn IJ, Murdock PR, Holbrook JD, Plumpton C, Macphee CH, Smith SA. Resistin is expressed in human macrophages and directly regulated by PPAR gamma activators. Biochemical and Biophysical Research Communications. 2003;**300**(2):472-476. DOI: https://doi.org/10.1016/S0006-291X(02)02841-3

[167] Badoer E, Kosari S, Stebbing MJ. Resistin, an adipokine with non-generalized actions on sympathetic nerve activity. Frontiers in Physiology. 2015;**6**:321. DOI: 10.3389/fphys.2015.00321

[168] Lee JH, Chan JL, Yiannakouris N, Kontogianni M, Estrada E, Seip R, Orlova C, Mantzoros CS. Circulating resistin levels are not associated with obesity or insulin resistance in humans and are not regulated by fasting or leptin administration: Cross-sectional and interventional studies in normal, insulin-resistant, and diabetic subjects. The Journal of Clinical Endocrinology and Metabolism. 2003;**88**(10):4848-4856. DOI: 10.1210/jc.2003-030519

[169] Silha JV, Krsek M, Skrha JV, Sucharda P, Nyomba BL, Murphy LJ. Plasma resistin, adiponectin and leptin levels in lean and obese subjects: Correlations with insulin resistence. European Journal of Endocrinology. 2003;**149**(4):331-335. PMID: 14514348

[170] Nogueiras R, Gallego R, Gualillo O, Caminos JE, García-Caballero T, Casanueva FF, Diéguez C. Resistin is expressed in different rat tissues and is regulated in a tissue- and gender-specific manner. FEBS Letters. 2003;**548**(1-3):21-27. DOI: 10.1016/S0014-5793(03)00708-7

[171] Huang SW, Seow KM, Ho LT, Chien Y, Chung DY, Chang CL, Lai YH, Hwang JL, Juan CC. Resistin mRNA levels are downregulated by estrogen in vivo and in vitro. FEBS Letters. 2005;**579**(2):449-454. DOI: 10.1016/j.febslet.2004.12.010

[172] Morash BA, Willkinson D, Ur E, Wilkinson M. Resistin expression and regulation in mouse pituitary. FEBS Letters. 2002;**526**(1-3):26-30. DOI: 10.1016/S0014-5793(02)03108-3

[173] Morash BA, Ur E, Wiesner G, Roy J, Wilkinson M. Pituitary resistin gene expression: Effects of age, gender and obesity. Neuroendocrinology. 2004;**79**(3):149-156. DOI: 10.1159/000077273

[174] Sarmento-Cabral A, Peinado JR, Halliday LC, Malagon MM, Castaño JP, Kineman RD, Luque RM. Adipokines (leptin, adiponectin, resistin) differentially regulate all hormonal cell types in primary anterior pituitary cell cultures from two primate species. Scientific Reports. 2017;**7**:43537. DOI: 10.1038/srep43537

[175] Benomar Y, Amine H, Crépin D, Al Rifai S, Riffault L, Gertler A, Taouis M. Central resistin/TLR4 impairs adiponectin signaling, contributing to insulin and FGF21 resistance. Diabetes. 2016;**65**(4):913-926. DOI: 10.2337/db15-1029

Chapter 3

The Biological Role of Androgen Receptor in Prostate Cancer Progression

Ken-ichi Takayama

Additional information is available at the end of the chapter

http://dx.doi.org/10.5772/intechopen.76360

Abstract

Prostate cancer is the most commonly diagnosed cancer in men all over the world. Localized cancers in the early stages can be well managed by surgical or radiation therapy. Metastatic prostate cancer is treated with androgen deprivation therapy because androgen signaling is essential to the prostate tumor growth and anti-apoptotic ability. However, resistance develops quickly in the clinical course and leads to castration-resistant prostate cancer (CRPC). Androgen receptor (AR) functions as a nuclear receptor to facilitate ligand-dependent transcriptional activation in the nucleus. AR interacts with several tissue-specific transcription factors such as forkhead box protein A1 (FOXA1) and regulates epigenetic status by recruiting epigenetic factors. In addition, AR transcriptional activity is modulated by interacting directly or indirectly with non-coding RNAs such as long non-coding RNAs (lncRNAs) and micro RNAs (miRNAs). Notably, enhanced AR signaling in CRPC has been documented in several studies; however, which of these factors are important for the biological function it remains poorly understood. Here, I review our current knowledge of the mechanistic roles of AR involved in prostate cancer progression and discuss the importance of the prostate cancer-associated signals.

Keywords: androgen receptor, prostate cancer, non-coding RNA, transcription, epigenetic

1. Introduction

Released hormone to an entire body is responsible for the development of various human diseases and physiology. Androgens, male sex hormones, mediate their effects predominantly by binding to the androgen receptor (AR), a member of the ligand-dependent nuclear receptor superfamily. Two major androgens, testosterone and dihydrotestosterone (DHT), bind and activate

AR to regulate target gene expression [1]. Testosterone produced in the testes is the most abundant androgen. After diffusing into cells, testosterone is converted to dihydrotestosterone (DHT) by the enzyme 5α-reductase [2]. DHT directly binds to and activates AR even more tightly than testosterone [3]. Androgens play a key role in the development of the male genital tract favoring differentiation and external genitalia during fetal life and sexual characteristic during puberty and are required for the establishment of adult sexual function. In addition to the classical activities in the male reproductive system, androgens also have anabolic functions in other tissues such as bone, muscle and central nervous systems [4]. Notably, AR has a central role in prostate cancer progression. In this review, we focus on AR functions through epigenetic factors and non-coding RNAs that have been shown to play a role in prostate cancer progression.

2. De-regulation of AR during the progression of prostate cancer

AR is a member of the nuclear receptor superfamily [5] and plays a key role in androgen signaling (**Figure 1A**). In the absence of ligand, AR is expressed mainly in the cytoplasm forming a complex with molecular chaperones and co-chaperones from the heat shock protein (Hsp) family. Upon androgen treatment, a conformational change in the complex leads to nuclear translocation of AR. In the nucleus, AR binds as a dimer to specific DNA sequences called androgen responsive elements (AREs), which are found in the vicinity of AR target genes [6]. AR activates gene expressions by modifying the epigenetic condition of AR binding regions [7]. Generally, nuclear receptors including AR have multiple domains called DNA binding domain, a ligand-binding domain (LBD), and an N-terminal domain (NTD), [2, 8, 9]. In the NTD, the transcriptional activation function 1 (AF1) domain promotes transcriptional activation with or without ligand binding [10], which is associated with enhanced AR function. AF2 domain in the LBD interacts with co-regulators with LXXLL motif [3]. Point mutations mapped to the LBD have been identified to have relevance with the treatment-resistance to drugs targeting AR in prostate cancer [11, 12].

Prostate cancer is one of the leading causes of cancer morbidity and mortality in developed countries. Androgens induce proliferation of prostate epithelial cells or prostate cancer tumor growth [13]. Early diagnosis of prostate cancer is currently based on the measurement of serum prostate-specific antigen (PSA), a representative AR target gene. Treatment of localized prostate cancer is determined based on clinico-pathological factors such as Gleason score, initial PSA level, patient's age and clinical tumor stage [14]. Because AR and its downstream signaling are essential for the development and progression of both localized and advanced metastatic prostate cancer, hormone therapy is a first-line and initially successful strategy for treating advanced prostate cancer. Androgen deprivation therapy decreases the circulating testosterone levels to a very low amount, a condition called chemical castration of men [15].

However, most of these tumors relapse and progress to hormone therapy resistant prostate cancer (HRPC) or castration-resistant prostate cancer (CRPC). To overcome CRPC/HRPC, new AR inhibitors have been developed. Abiraterone acetate, a potent inhibitor of CYP17 reduces testosterone synthesis from cholesterol [16]. Despite suppression of circulating testosterone, castration does not decrease androgens enough from the prostate tumor microenvironment and residual androgen levels are well within the range capable of activating AR. Accordingly,

http://dx.doi.org/10.5772/intechopen.76360

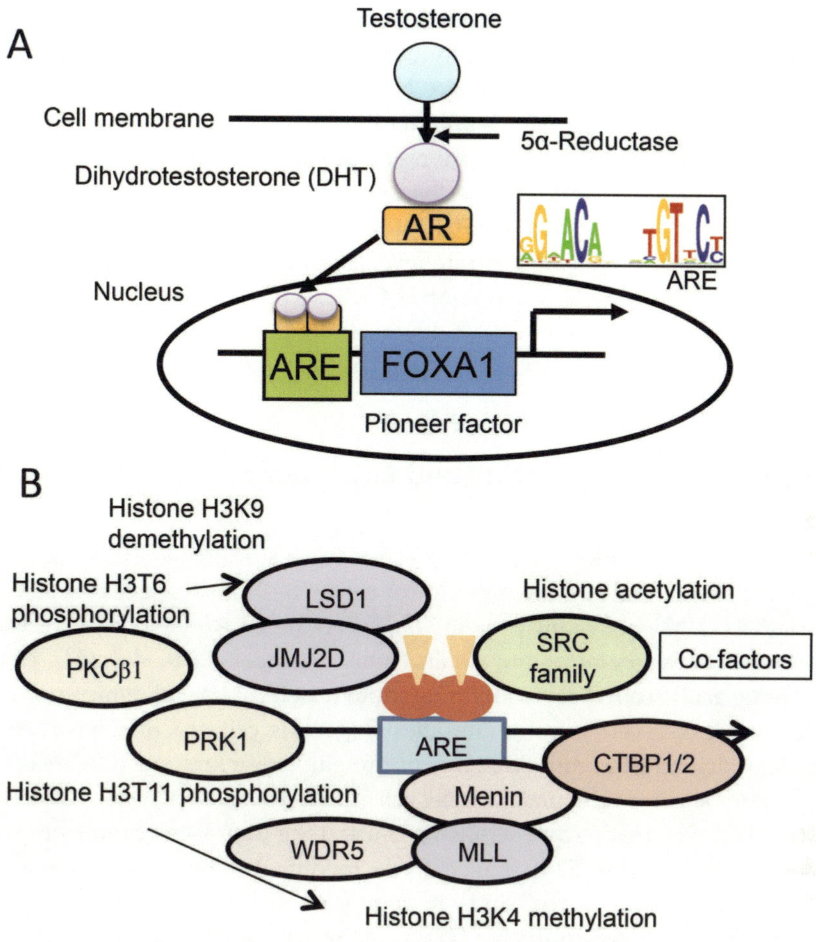

Figure 1. Epigenetic regulation of AR binding regions. (A) Androgen receptor (AR) translocates into the nucleus. By collaborating with FOXA1, AR is recruited to specific loci called androgen responsive elements (AREs) to activate its target genes. (B) Upon androgen treatment, several histone modifying enzymes were recruited to AR binding sites. PKCβ1-mediated histone H3T6 phosphorylation directs LSD1 for not H3K4 but H3K9 demethylation by cooperating with JMJ2D. H3T11 phosphorylation also accelerates WDR5-mediated MLL recruitments and LSD1 activity. MLL complex interacts with AR through menin and promotes histone H3K4 methylation to enhance AR dependent gene expression. SRC family and CTBP1/2 are AR interacting cofactors for histone acetylation or deacetylation.

therapeutic strategies effectively targeting production of intratumoral androgens are necessary. Clinical studies showed that abiraterone improved overall survival, progression free survival, delayed initiation of chemotherapy and doubled the time to first skeletal event. Enzalutamide (MDV3100) is another novel endocrine treatment with reported significant anti-tumor activity [17]. It is an AR-receptor-signaling inhibitor, blocking nuclear translocation, DNA binding, and co-activator recruitment. Enzalutamide significantly prolonged the survival of men with metastatic CRPC after chemotherapy [18]. Although these new types of drugs bring impressive results, the duration of response is variable, and a majority eventually progress with a rising PSA. While the mechanisms determining resistance have not been fully elucidated, persistent AR activation provides a compelling rationale for developing more strategies to inhibit AR [19].

Enhanced AR downstream signals are caused by AR gene amplification, point mutation, AR variants (particularly AR-Vs), hypersensitivity to androgens, or intratumoral steroidogenesis [20–23]. AR mRNA is alternatively spliced to AR-Vs and results in prematurely termination of the full AR protein. Most AR-Vs are missing LBD, however, retain the NTD to drive transcription androgen-independently. Among these variants, AR-V7 is expressed in HRPC/CRPCs most frequently and could be the therapeutic target of tumors resistant to existing therapies directed to androgen/AR [24, 25]. In addition, elevated AR expression increased the reactivity of prostate cancer cells to castrate levels of androgens and promotes resistance to AR-targeting drugs. Increased AR expression in CRPC is often mediated by AR gene amplification. Thus, it is critical to investigate AR downstream-signaling or regulatory mechanisms by AR to understand how CRPC develop among the patients.

3. Investigation of AR-regulators and target genes

Chromatin immunoprecipitation (ChIP) and sequencing studies have revealed locations of AR bindings have been found in prostate cancer cells [26–28]. AR target genes such as ADP-ribosylation factor GTPase-activating protein 3 (ARFGAP3) [29], Amyloid Beta Precursor Protein (APP) [30], Acyl-CoA Synthetase Long Chain Family Member 3 (ACSL3) [31], claudin-8 [32] and Transforming acidic coiled-coil-containing protein 2 (TACC2) [33], which promotes tumor growth by regulating cell cycle, intratumoral steroidogenesis, cell structure, have been identified in my research. Calcium/calmodulin-dependent protein kinase kinase 2 (CAMKK2) is overexpressed in prostate cancer and regulates cancer cell growth via its unexpected role as a hormone-dependent modulator of anabolic metabolism, contributing to prostate cancer progression [26]. Ubiquitin-conjugating enzyme E2 C (UBE2C) was identified to be a CRPC-specific AR target gene and promoted G2/M mitotic cell division in prostate cancer cells [27]. Interestingly, androgen regulates p53 localization by inducing GTPase-activating protein-binding protein 2 (G3BP2), which is an AR target gene [34]. G3BP2 associates with p53 and SUMO E3 ligase RAN binding protein 2 (RanBP2), promoting p53 nuclear export via increased p53 sumoylation. Elevated G3BP2 expression repressed docetaxel-mediated apoptosis and promoted CRPC tumor growth.

3.1. Epigenetic factors

In prostate cancer, deregulation of AR interaction with its coregulators within nucleus is common and activation of coregulators is frequently observed. AR has a role in the ligand-dependent epigenetic changes by interacting with various coregulators such as histone-modifying enzymes. DNA, histones and other proteins formed chromatin as a highly ordered structure. Chromatin forms a unit called the nucleosome consisting of a histone octamer (H2A, H2B, H3 and H4, two pairs of each) and DNA. Both DNA methylation and histone modification patterns have also been investigated in prostate cancer. Histone modifications affect the interaction of DNA with histones, transcription factors or other proteins binding to DNA, thus playing a role in the epigenetic control of biological events. Lysine, arginine, serine and threonine residues enriched in N-terminal histone tails serve as substrates for post-translational modifications such as acetylation, phosphorylation, methylation, ubiquitination, sumoylation and deamination. Histone H3, one of the major histones, is most representative for epigenetic regulation. The methylation of lysine on position 9 (H3K9) and H3K27 is an epigenetic mark of condensed chromatin and silent loci. The methylation of H3K4 and H3K36 is associated with open chromatin structures. Acetylation of lysine residues of H3 is also correlated with enhanced enhancer/promoter activation. [5].

In a recent report, the potential for BET bromodomain protein inhibitors as a novel epigenetic approach to treatment of CRPC has been shown [35]. In prostate cancer cell lines, BET bromodomain inhibitor, JQ1, was demonstrated to induce apoptosis and down-regulate AR target gene expression. Bromodomain and the extra-terminal (BET) subfamily of human bromodomain proteins (BRDs), with a focus on BRD4, were found to play a major role in AR signaling and interact with AR via bromodomain 1/2. JQ1 inhibits this BRD4-AR bond, resulting in removal of RNA polymerase II from AR target genes [35]. This study suggests for the first time that modulating epigenetic function of AR could be a useful strategy to overcome clinical problems associated with AR signals.

Histone acetylation loosens the nucleosome packing within chromatin to increase DNA accessibility, resulting in the recruitment of chromatin remodeling factors that lead to enhanced transcriptional activity. The BRD has the ability to recognize acetylated lysine residues [36]. This activity allows BRDs to play a vital role in histone acetylation-mediated gene transcriptional regulation in chromatin. Such BRDs included Tripartite motif containing 24 (TRIM24), which interacts with AR and are highly expressed in CRPC [37]. Other studies revealed that E3 ubiquitin ligase substrate binding adaptor speckle-type POZ protein (SPOP) binds to and induces ubiquitination of BRD4 for degradation. In many prostate cancer tissues, SPOP is the most frequently mutated to enhance the expression level of BRD4 [38].

AR regulates the histone modifications in AR binding sites (ARBSs) and promotes enhancer activity by directly interacting with many co-regulators including steroid receptor coactivators (SRCs) or other histone-modifying enzymes [6, 39] (**Figure 1B**). Methylations of H3K4 (mono-, di- or tri-methylation) indicate the active promoter/enhancer regions [40] and promoted by the SET1/MLL histone methyltransferase (HMTase) complex. Menin protein binding to the N-terminus of MLL is important for MLL target gene expressions. Menin directly binds to AR and recruited MLL complex. Menin is highly expressed in CRPC tissues and associated with castration-resistant tumor growth [41]. Importantly, small molecule inhibitors against menin-MLL interaction could be the new useful drugs for CRPC. MLL complex plays an important role for androgen-mediated gene induction and its activity is regulated finely. After androgen stimulation, protein kinase C-related kinase 1 (PRK1) promotes histone H3 threonine 11 phosphorylation (H3T11P) [42]. WD repeat containing protein 5 (WDR5), a subunit of the SET1/MLL complex, associates with H3T11P and then promotes the recruitment of the MLL complex for H3K4 tri-methylation (H3K4me3) in ARBSs [43]. WDR5 is a critical epigenetic integrator and is overexpressed in prostate cancers. PRK1 kinase activity facilitates demethylation of H3K9 by cooperating with lysine-specific demethylase 1 (LSD1) [42, 44]. In addition, Protein kinase C beta 1 (PKCβ1) phosphorylates histone H3T6 to prevent lysine specific demethylase including LSD1 from histone H3K4 demethylation [45]. Moreover, C-terminal binding protein 2 (CTBP2) is an androgen-responsive cofactor of AR. CTBP2 repressed tumor-suppressor genes and AR corepressors in prostate cancer cells, such as Nuclear receptor co-repressor (NCOR) and receptor-interacting protein 140 (RIP140), by binding with AR to the promoter enhancers of these genes. Moreover, global gene-expression analyses revealed a positive effect on androgen-mediated gene expression, and CTBP2 silencing was found to increase AR interactions with corepressors that limit histone modification [46]. Thus, these findings have a clinical relevance to develop new drugs for treatment by regulating epigenetic status [41].

Histone modification is also important for increased AR expression in CRPC [47]. Recent studies showed that both transcriptional and epigenetic changes are important for AR upregulation in prostate cancer. To introns of the AR gene, recruitments of AR and its associated cofactors such as LSD1, which represses transcription by inhibiting histone H3K4 methylation are induced by androgen. This feedback loop mechanism regulates AR expression negatively by androgen. Interestingly, after long-term incubation in castration level of androgens, AR expression increases in prostate cancer cells and then low levels of androgens can activate AR regulated genes in CRPC without repressing genes such as the AR itself.

3.2. Collaborative transcription factors

Functional ARBSs were not only determined by sequence motifs but also chromatin accessibility. ChIP-sequence (ChIP-seq) analyses using next-generation sequencers have been developed as a high-throughput strategy to identify transcription factor binding regions [48]. For instance, AR ChIP-seq was performed in two LNCaP-derived prostate cancer cell lines with higher AR expression [49]. Interestingly, more ARBSs were obtained in these cell lines when they were treated with low concentrations of androgen. These data indicate that the higher expression of AR sensitizes the receptor binding to genome, thus illustrating the mechanism that the AR signaling pathway is enhanced in CRPC.

Furthermore, by analyzing enriched motifs around ARBSs, AR-associated transcription partners such as forkhead box protein A1 (FOXA1) [50], ERG, GATA2 [51], Oct1 [31], RUNX1 [52] and NKX3–1 [50] have been mapped to the prostate cancer genome and these studies suggested the global role of these factor to activate AR-driven transcriptional program. Among them, a chromatin-opening transcription factor, FOXA1, is able to directly bind to the chromatin to open up the local nucleosomal domain (**Figure 1A**). In prostate cells, FOXA1 protein has been shown physically interact with the AR protein and plays critical roles in regulating the transcription of prostate genes [7]. Moreover, ARBSs in CRPC tissues were found by ChIP-seq and most of them could not been identified in cell lines. Many adjacent genes were *in vivo* restricted set of AR-regulated genes. Transcription factor motifs such as E2F, Myc and STAT were significantly enriched in these CRPC-specific ARBSs [53]. Another study revealed the colocalization of FOXA1 and homeobox B13 (HOXB13) at a set of ARBSs in human tumor tissues. These ARBSs were consistently reprogrammed for prostate tumor development [54].

4. The roles of non-coding RNAs in AR action and prostate cancer biology

Recent advances in DNA sequence technology have demonstrated that more than 90% of the human genome is actively transcribed. The encyclopedia of DNA elements (ENCODE) project has shown that only 2% of these transcripts are translated into proteins [55]. The non-coding RNAs (ncRNAs), that occupy the majority of transcripts in the nucleus, were initially thought as the "dark matter." Non-coding RNAs are broadly categorized into short and long transcripts. Short non-coding RNAs with a length within 200 nucleotides include such as transfer RNA, microRNA (miRNA), and snoRNA. miRNAs play important roles in cancer by post-transcriptional modification of target mRNA or protein expression. Long non-coding RNAs (lncRNAs) represent most of the transcribed ncRNA in the human genome longer than 200 bp. GENCODE v27 includes 15,778 human lncRNA-related genes, which produce 27,908 lncRNAs [56].

4.1. lncRNA

LncRNAs exhibit similar structure and biogenesis as mRNAs. They are polyadenylated and may function in either nuclear or cytoplasmic compartments. Growing number of evidences have shown that lncRNAs are involved in numerous human diseases including cancer [57]. Global nuclear run-on sequencing (GRO-seq) was developed as a new technology to detect androgen-induced transcripts including lncRNAs [58]. This study has demonstrated that the production of enhancer-templated non-coding RNAs (eRNAs) is important for nucleosome remodeling to induce enhancer/promoter interaction by looping and gene activation. It was also shown that androgen promotes both transcriptional initiation and elongation. These active enhancers are tuned dynamically to modulate gene expression network in prostate cancer. AR is widely recruited to these eRNA-bound enhancer- promoter regions for activating the genes in the vicinity. Interestingly, knockdown of eRNA represses androgen-dependent enhancer promoter interaction and gene activation [59]. DNA nicking activity of topoisomerase I (TOP1) was found to produce robust eRNA for enhancer activation. Furthermore, DNA damage repair machinery is recruited kinetically to the AR-regulated enhancers [60].

LncRNAs are able to fold into secondary and tertiary structures by which they perform their function (**Figure 2A**). Direct regulation of AR epigenetic function by lncRNA is strikingly receiving attention among all. *Prostate cancer gene expression marker 1* (*PCGEM1*) was found as an androgen-regulated and prostate tissue-specific lncRNA [61]. Overexpression of *PCGEM1* in prostate tumors were observed and associated with the anti-apoptotic activity by inhibiting p53 and p21 induction [62]. *Prostate cancer noncoding RNA 1* (*PRNCR1*) was identified by investigating the surrounding region of SNPs (single nucleotide polymorphisms) correlated with prostate cancer susceptibility. Importantly, both *PCGEM1* and *PRNCR1* cooperatively functions for AR-mediated gene expression [63]. The association of *PCGEM1* and *PRNCR1* with AR was shown to be essential in the process of AR activation. Moreover, *PCGEM1* was found to interact with pygopus homolog2 (Pygo2) and *PRNCR1* with DOT1-like histone H3 methyltransferase (DOT1L). By modulating AR proteins with such interacted enzymes, these two lncRNAs were shown to be responsible for AR-associated loop formation between enhancer and promoter.

Another lncRNA, *steroid receptor RNA activator* (*SRA*) modulates the functions of various nuclear receptors, such as AR, estrogen receptor (ER), progesterone receptor (PR), glucocorticoid receptor (GR) and thyroid hormone receptor (TR). *SRA* associates with a coactivator SRC-1 (steroid receptor coactivator) and six stem-loop motifs in *SRA* are required for co-activation. Interestingly, overexpression of *SRA* was found in various tumors including prostate cancer compared with normal tissues [64, 65].

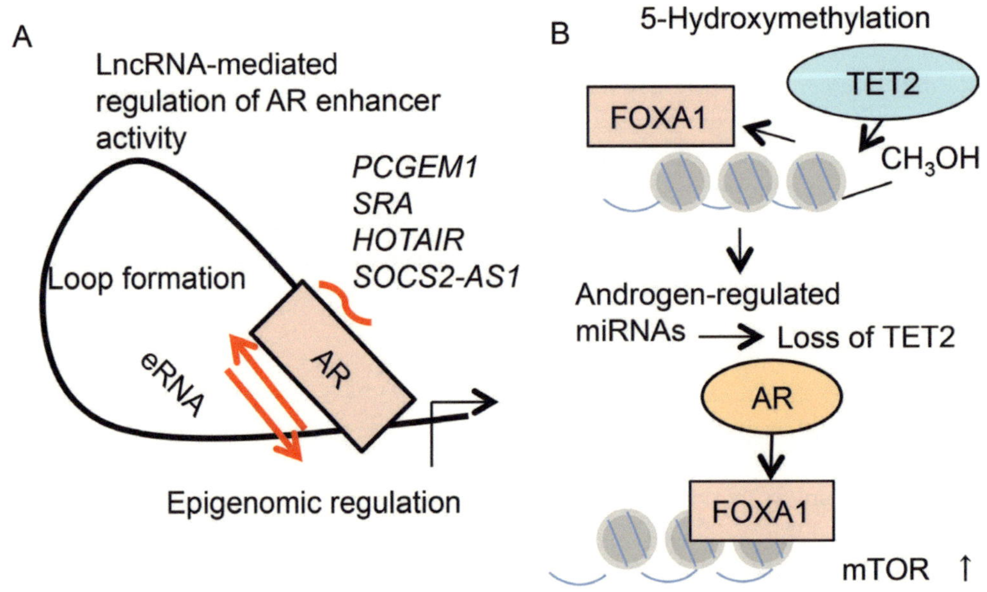

Figure 2. The role of non-coding RNA in AR-mediated transcription. (A) The role of enhancer RNA (eRNA) or other AR interacting lncRNAs. These lncRNAs (eRNA, *PCGEM1, PRNCR1 or SRA*) promotes loop formation for promoter/enhancer interaction. *HOTAIR* enhances AR protein stability by inhibiting ubiquitylation of AR. *SOCS2-AS1* regulates cofactor recruitments to AR. (B) Androgen-induced miRNA mediated TET2 repression inhibits 5-hmC modifications in FOXA1 occupied enhancer regions. By removal of 5-hmC, FOXA1 is activated and induce FOXA1 or ARregulated genes such as mTOR.

HOX Antisense Intergenic RNA (*HOTAIR*) is an lncRNA transcribed in the antisense direction from the *HOXC* gene cluster. *HOTAIR* associates with the polycomb repressive complex 2 (PRC2) for acting as a transcriptional regulators in trans. PRC2 is recruited to the HOXD locus *HOTAIR*-dependently, leading to silenced transcription across a 40-kb region. Moreover, *HOTAIR* associates with LSD1/CoREST/REST complex. This interaction coupled PRC2 and LSD1 to induce histone H3K27 methylation and K4 demethylation for gene silencing [66]. Thus, lncRNAs interacts with chromatin remodeling complexes to promote heterochromatin formation in specific loci, resulting in target gene expression changes. In addition, *HOTAIR* expression is correlated with the disease progressions of breast and prostate cancer [67, 68]. *HOTAIR* high expressions in these cancers are correlated with poor prognosis. This finding reflects the regulation of steroid hormone function by *HOTAIR*. *HOTAIR* is negatively regulated by androgen treatment and induced by depleting androgen. Mechanistically, *HOTAIR* blocks the association of E3-ubiquitine ligase MDM2 with AR by binding to AR. This binding inhibits ubiquitin-mediated degradation and stabilizes AR protein level to activate the AR mediated transcription for driving CRPC development [68].

Suppressor of cytokine signaling 2-antisense transcript 1 (*SOCS2-AS1*) was found in our directional RNA-seq and ChIP-seq analysis [69]. *SOCS2-AS1* is highly expressed in castration-resistant model cells and promotes cell proliferation and inhibits apoptosis induced by docetaxel. *SOCS2-AS1* repressed apoptosis-related genes such as TNFSF10/TRAIL, which are AR target genes. For molecular mechanism in this gene regulation, *SOCS2-AS1* is involved with AR activation by promoting the recruitments of coregulators to AR-occupied regions by interacting with AR (**Figure 2A**).

Global transcriptome analysis showed that most of the genome can be transcribed from both sense and antisense strands. More than 1000 pairs of sense/antisense transcripts were obtained and antisense transcription is involved in such bidirectional gene regulation [70, 71]. Sense-transcript is regulated by antisense through several mechanisms. For example, post-transcriptional degradation is caused by antisense transcript. Another mechanism is recruitments of antisense RNA associated transcription factors for epigenetic regulation. In prostate cancer, an lncRNA, *Prostate cancer antigen 3* (*PCA3*), was found to be an overexpressed in prostate cancer tissues. In 95% of the prostate tumors, the expression of *PCA3* is upregulated compared with adjacent normal prostate tissues. *PCA3* RNA levels can also be measured by urinary test more specifically than prostate specific antigen (PSA) measurement [72]. Therefore, it can be a helpful biomarker to diagnose prostate cancer [73]. AS an antisense transcript, *PCA3* functions as an oncogenic lncRNA by inhibiting its overlapped gene Prune Homolog 2 (PRUNE2), which is a tumor suppressor gene. *PCA3* represses *PRUNE2* expression by formation of a double-stranded RNA with *PRUNE2* mRNA for reducing post transcriptionally [74].

Genome-wide androgen-regulated transcriptome analysis identified a new androgen-responsive lncRNA, *CTBP1-AS* [75]. C-terminal binding protein 1 (CTBP1) functions as a transcriptional repressor for AR and negatively regulates AR downstream signals. It was demonstrated that *CTBP1-AS* is regulated by AR-bindings to its promoter region. In addition, *CTBP1-AS* associates with a RNA binding protein, PSF (PTB-associated splicing factor) to transcriptionally repress its target genes such as CTBP1 via histone deacetylation [75]. Then androgen-regulated lncRNAs mediates AR function by modulating epigenetic status and gene expression. Moreover, *CTBP1-AS* promotes prostate cancer cell cycle progression by repressing cell cycle regulators such as p53 and SMAD3 globally [75]. Thus, *CTBP1-AS* and PSF modulate global gene expression transcriptionally and post-transcriptionally to promote AR and prostate cancer-associated signals. These findings suggest that targeting *CTBP1-AS* and PSF may represent a useful therapeutic strategy to overcome castration-resistance in prostate cancer.

Interestingly, another report has shown that PSF binds to another CRPC-associated lncRNA, *Second Chromosome Locus Associated with Prostate 1* (*SChLAP1*) [76], and mRNAs of various AR target genes to enhance their stability. In CRPC model cells, pathway analysis showed that PSF primarily targets spliceosome genes for enhancing their expressions. Interestingly, in addition to PSF, these wide-range of spliceosome genes are overexpressed in metastatic prostate cancer tissues, suggesting the importance of splicing factors in the disease progression. PSF also binds to *AR* mRNA promoting AR splicing such as AR-V7 and expression [76] in CRPC. In addition to PSF, heterogeneous nuclear ribonucleoprotein L (HNRNPL) was identified by CRISPR/Cas9 knockout screen to be required for prostate cancer growth. HNRNPL also regulates the alternative splicing of a set of RNAs, including *AR* transcript [77]. Collectively, these recent studies revealed the novel roles of RNA processing factors in modulation of AR splicing and expression. Aberrant expressions of splicing factors would induce the diversity of oncogenic gene expressions for promoting prostate cancer.

Growth arrest-specific 5 (*GAS5*) was originally identified as a gene that is preferentially expressed in growth arrested cells [78]. In prostate cancer cell lines, overexpression of *GAS5* induced apoptosis [79] and cell cycle arrest via enhanced expression of p27, a tumor suppressor [80]. *GAS5* associates with steroid receptors including AR and forms a structure that blocks the DNA-binding site of the steroid receptor, resulting in repression of steroid-mediated transcription [81].

These analyses of lncRNA functions revealed a novel transcriptional regulatory mechanism. Several lncRNAs such as *SRA* and *SOCS2-AS1* associate with AR protein and promote recruitment of cofactors (**Figure 2A**). Other mechanisms contain loop forming between promoter and enhancer (eRNA, *PCGEM1* and *PRNCR1*) or enhancing AR protein stability (*HOTAIR*) to activate AR action. Regulation of genes related with cancer development or cell cycle controls by interacting with RNA-binding transcriptional repressor (*CTBP1-AS*) would be another mechanism to promote cancer progression. Androgen-regulated lncRNAs (*PCGEM1*, *HOTAIR*, *CTBP1-AS* and *SOCS2-AS1*) have important roles in these gene expressions. Moreover, recent analyses have shown the importance of RNA-binding proteins (PSF/NONO, HNRNPL) in prostate cancer progression. Because only a limited number of lncRNA functions have been demonstrated, we should investigate molecular functions of more lncRNAs in tissue and spatial specific manner in the future.

4.2. miRNA

MicroRNAs (miRNAs) are evolutionally conserved single-stranded small non-protein Generally miRNAs binds to the 3′ untranslated region (UTR) of mRNAs to inhibit their translation. For examples, dysregulation of miRNA expression profiles during the progression of prostate cancer have been discussed [82]. In these studies, miR-21, miR-29a/b, miR-32, miR-99a, miR-148a, miR-125b and miR-141 were found to be androgen-regulated miRNAs and dysregulated in prostate cancer. Upregulated miR-21 enhanced AR-dependent cell proliferation and associated with development of CRPC [83, 84]. Another androgen regulated miRNA, miR-125b targets apoptosis inducing factors regulated by p53 (PUMA and BAK1) [85]. Thus, by repressing these genes, overexpression of miR-125b in tumors collapses the balance between pro- and anti-apoptotic processes. It was shown that miR-148a is also regulated by androgen and highly induced in AR positive prostate cancer cells. miR-148a targets cullin-associated and neddylation dissociated 1 (CAND1), a cell cycle regulator, to promote cell proliferation [86]. Moreover, miR-32 inhibits apoptosis by targeting BIM, a pro-apoptotic member of the BCL2 family [87]. Both miR-32 and miR-148a were overexpressed in CRPC tissues, indicating that these miRNAs have important roles in the promotion of castration-resistance [87].

DNA methylation is also the representative epigenetic mark adding a methyl group to the 5′ position of cytosine (5-mC). DNA methylation is added or removed in a spatially and temporally defined context throughout the genome including enhancer/promoter regions. DNA methyltransferases (DNMTs) contributes to the process as enzymes. DNMTs include DNMT3A/DNMT3B for de novo and DNMT1 for maintenance of methylation. The ten-eleven translocation (TET) family proteins catalyzed the production of 5-hydroxymethylcytosine (5-hmC), an oxidation product of 5-mC. Several studies have demonstrated that 5-hmC is not only an intermediate product of a demethylation process, but can also function as a stable epigenetic mark [88].

Interestingly, recent study has demonstrated that miR-29 family and miR-22 are highly induced by androgen in hormone-therapy resistant prostate cancer [89]. In prostate cancer clinical samples revealed that the expression level of miR-29a/b is negatively associated with that of TET2. Interestingly, *in situ* hybridization (ISH) study of clinical samples indicated that miR-29a/b is highly expressed in a subset of prostate cancers with poor prognoses. Mechanistically, TET2 repression decreased 5-hmC levels, which is correlated with FOXA1 transcriptional activity. FOXA1 activation induced expressions of prostate cancer related genes. One of such 5-hmC regulated genes was mammalian target of rapamycin (mTOR) (**Figure 2B**). These experimental and clinical data suggested a novel oncogenic role of miR-29 family in prostate cancer progression [89]. The roles of miR-29 family in cancer are still controversial because their expressions are reduced in several cancer tissues in comparison with normal [90]. However, their overexpression inhibits apoptosis in lung cancer as oncogenic miRNAs [91]. Exome sequencing analysis revealed that somatic mutations of TET2 exon are involved in metastatic CRPC development [92]. Rare variation in TET2 is also associated with the development of prostate cancer [93]. TET2 could directly regulate AR-signaling by binding to AR [94]. Thus, the role of TET2 and 5-hmC-modification in prostate cancer deserves additional analysis and may define a subset of metastatic disease.

Studies of non-coding RNAs in AR signals are mainly reported in the research field of prostate cancer. However, knockout of the miRNA processing enzyme, Dicer 1, Ribonuclease III (DICER), in mice inhibited AR function tissue specifically in muscle. In addition, castration in rats inhibited the expression of a large set of miRNAs in prostate and muscle, suggesting the importance of miRNAs in the physiological functions of androgens in other tissues [95].

5. Conclusion and perspective

The majority of prostate cancer and CRPC tumors are driven by AR signaling. AR-mediated resistance to hormone therapy can be acquired by multiple mechanisms. AR mutation, amplification and truncated variants have been identified to explain aberrant AR activation in prostate cancer progression. AR coregulators and collaborating transcription factors are essentials for AR to exert its transcriptional activity. Recently the role of non-coding RNAs such as lncRNAs and miRNAs has been realized to play a critical role in AR activation and prostate cancer progression. Such alterations of AR function lead to positive or negative regulation of the growth and invasion ability of cancer cells. Although AR-targeting drugs have been developed, we could not eliminate CRPC due to the adaptive evolution of the disease during the treatment. Combinational therapies are required to overcome CRPC problems. Therefore, it is urgent to find better predictive biomarkers or therapeutic targets which have an efficacy for diagnosing and treating prostate cancer and CRPC.

Acknowledgements

This work was supported by grants from the JSPS (number 17H04334), Japan; grants from Takeda Science Foundation, Japan.

Conflict of interest

The author declares no conflict of interest.

Author details

Ken-ichi Takayama[1,2*]

*Address all correspondence to: ktakayama-tky@umin.ac.jp

1 Department of Functional Biogerontology, Tokyo Metropolitan Institute of Gerontology, Tokyo, Japan

2 Department of Geriatric Medicine, The University of Tokyo, Tokyo, Japan

References

[1] Takayama K, Inoue S. Transcriptional network of androgen receptor in prostate cancer progression. International Journal of Urology. 2013;**20**(8):756-768. DOI: 10.1111/iju.12146

[2] Heemers HV, Tindall DJ. Androgen receptor (AR) coregulators: A diversity of functions converging on and regulating the AR transcriptional complex. Endocrine Reviews. 2007;**28**:778-808. DOI: 10.1210/er.2007-0019

[3] Heery DM, Kalkhoven E, Hoare S, Parker MG. A signature motif in transcriptional coactivatorsmediates binding to nuclear receptors. Nature. 1997;**387**:733-736. DOI: 10.1038/42750

[4] Ophoff J, Callewaert F, Venken K, De Gendt K, Ohlsson C, Gayan-Ramirez G, et al. Physical activity in the androgen receptor knockout mouse: Evidence for reversal of androgen deficiency on cancellous bone. Biochemical and Biophysical Research Communications. 2009;**378**(1):139-144. DOI: 10.1016/j.bbrc.2008.11.016

[5] Dasgupta S. Nuclear receptor coactivators: Master regulators of human health and disease. Annual Review of Medicine. 2014;**65**:279-292

[6] Shang Y, Myers M, Brown M. Formation of the androgen receptor transcription complex. Molecular Cell. 2002;**9**:601-610

[7] Lupien M, Eeckhoute J, Meyer CA, Wang Q, Zhang Y, Li W, et al. FoxA1 translates epigenetic signatures into enhancer-driven lineage-specific transcription. Cell. 2008;**132**(6):958-970. DOI: 10.1016/j.cell.2008.01.018

[8] Jenster G, van der Korput HA, van Vroonhoven C, van der Kwast TH, Trapman J, Brinkmann AO. Domains of the human androgen receptor involved in steroid binding, transcriptional activation, and subcellular localization. Molecular Endocrinology. 1991;**5**:1396-1404. DOI: 10.1210/mend-5-10-1396

[9] Jenster G, van der Korput HA, Trapman J, Brinkmann AO. Identification of two transcription activation units in the N-terminal domain of the human androgen receptor. The Journal of Biological Chemistry. 1995;**270**:7341-7346

[10] Dehm SM, Regan KM, Schmidt LJ, Tindall DJ. Selective role of an NH_2-terminal WxxLF motif for aberrant androgen receptor activation in androgen depletion-independent prostate cancer cells. Cancer Research. 2007;**67**:10067-10077. DOI: 10.1158/0008-5472.CAN-07-1267

[11] Buchanan G, Greenberg NM, Scher HI, Harris JM, Marshall VR, Tilley WD. Collocation of androgen receptor gene mutations in prostate cancer. Clinical Cancer Research. 2001;**7**:1273-1281

[12] Taplin ME, Bubley GJ, Shuster TD, Frantz ME, Spooner AE, Ogata GK, Keer HN, Balk SP. Mutation of the androgen-receptor gene in metastatic androgen-independent prostate cancer. The New England Journal of Medicine. 1995;**332**:1393-1398. DOI: 10.1056/NEJM199505253322101

[13] La Vignera S, Condorelli RA, Russo GI, Morgia G, Calogero AE. Endocrine control of benign prostatic hyperplasia. Andrology. 2016;**4**(3):404-411. DOI: 10.1111/andr.12186

[14] Attard G, Parker C, Eeles RA, Schröder F, Tomlins SA, Tannock I, Drake CG, de Bono JS, et al. Prostate cancer. Lancet. 2016;**387**:70-82. DOI: 10.1016/S0140-6736(14)61947-4

[15] Bill-Axelson A, Holmberg L, Ruutu M, Garmo H, Stark JR, Busch C, et al. Radical prostatectomy or watchful waiting in early prostate cancer. The New England Journal of Medicine. 2014;**370**:932-942. DOI: 10.1056/NEJMoa1011967

[16] de Bono JS, Logothetis CJ, Molina A, Fizazi K, North S, Chu L, et al. Abiraterone and increased survival in metastatic prostate cancer. The New England Journal of Medicine. 2011;**364**:1995-2005. DOI: 10.1056/NEJMoa1014618

[17] Tran C, Ouk S, Clegg NJ, Chen Y, Watson PA, Arora V, et al. Development of a second-generation antiandrogen for treatment of advanced prostate cancer. Science. 2009;**324**:787-790. DOI: 10.1126/science.1168175

[18] Scher HI, Fizazi K, Saad F, Taplin ME, Sternberg CN, Miller K, et al. Increased survival with enzalutamide in prostate cancer after chemotherapy. The New England Journal of Medicine. 2012;**367**:1187-1197. DOI: 10.1056/NEJMoa1207506

[19] Elahe A. Mostaghel. Cancer Management and Research. 2014;**6**:39-51. DOI: 10.2147/CMAR.S39318

[20] Chen CD, Welsbie DS, Tran C, Baek SH, Chen R, Vessella R, Rosenfeld MG, Sawyers CL. Molecular determinants of resistance to antiandrogen therapy. Nature Medicine. 2004;**10**:33-39. DOI: 10.1038/nm972

[21] Locke JA, Guns ES, Lubik AA, Adomat HH, Hendy SC, Wood CA, et al. Androgen levels increase by intratumoral de novo steroidogenesis during progression of castration-resistant prostate cancer. Cancer Research. 2008;**68**:6407-6415. DOI: 10.1158/0008-5472.CAN-07-5997

[22] Sun S, Sprenger CC, Vessella RL, Haugk K, Soriano K, Mostaghel EA, et al. Castration resistance in human prostate cancer is conferred by a frequently occurring androgen receptor

splice variant. The Journal of Clinical Investigation. 2010;**120**:2715-2730. DOI: 10.1172/JCI41824

[23] Waltering KK, Helenius MA, Sahu B, Manni V, Linja MJ, Jänne OA, Visakorpi T. Increased expression of androgen receptor sensitizes prostate cancer cells to low levels of androgens. Cancer Research. 2009;**69**:8141-8149. DOI: 10.1158/0008-5472.CAN-09-0919

[24] Antonarakis ES, Lu C, Wang H, Luber B, Nakazawa M, Roeser JC, et al. AR-V7 and resistance to enzalutamide and abiraterone in prostate cancer. The New England Journal of Medicine. 2014;**371**:1028-1038. DOI: 10.1056/NEJMoa1315815

[25] Antonarakis ES, Armstrong AJ, Dehm SM, Luo J. Androgen receptor variant-driven prostate cancer: Clinical implications and therapeutic targeting. Prostate Cancer and Prostatic Diseases. 2016;**19**:231-241. DOI: 10.1038/pcan.2016.17

[26] Massie CE, Lynch A, Ramos-Montoya A, Boren J, Stark R, Fazli L, et al. The androgen receptor fuels prostate cancer by regulating central metabolism and biosynthesis. The EMBO Journal. 2011;**30**(13):2719-2733. DOI: 10.1038/emboj.2011.158

[27] Wang Q, Li W, Zhang Y, Yuan X, Xu K, Yu J, et al. Androgen receptor regulates a distinct transcription program in androgen-independent prostate cancer. Cell. 2009;**138**(2):245-256. DOI: 10.1016/j.cell.2009.04.056

[28] Sahu B, Laakso M, Ovaska K, Mirtti T, Lundin J, Rannikko A, et al. Dual role of FoxA1 in androgen receptor binding to chromatin, androgen signalling and prostate cancer. The EMBO Journal. 2011;**30**(19):3962-3976. DOI: 10.1038/emboj.2011.328

[29] Obinata D, Takayama K, Urano T, Murata T, Ikeda K, Horie-Inoue K, et al. ARFGAP3, an androgen target gene, promotes prostate cancer cell proliferation and migration. International Journal of Cancer. 2012;**130**(10):2240-2248. DOI: 10.1002/ijc.26224

[30] Takayama K, Tsutsumi S, Suzuki T, Horie-Inoue K, Ikeda K, Kaneshiro K, et al. Amyloid precursor protein is a primary androgen target gene that promotes prostate cancer growth. Cancer Research. 2009;**69**(1):137-142. DOI: 10.1158/0008-5472.CAN-08-3633

[31] Obinata D, Takayama K, Fujiwara K, Suzuki T, Tsutsumi S, Fukuda N, et al. Targeting Oct1 genomic function inhibits androgen receptor signaling and castration-resistant prostate cancer growth. Oncogene. 2016;**35**(49):6350-6358. DOI: 10.1038/onc.2016.171

[32] Ashikari D, Takayama KI, Obinata D, Takahashi S, Inoue S. CLDN8, an androgen-regulated gene, promotes prostate cancer cell proliferation and migration. Cancer Science. 2017;**108**(7):1386-1393. DOI: 10.1111/cas.13269

[33] Takayama K, Horie-Inoue K, Suzuki T, Urano T, Ikeda K, Fujimura T, et al. TACC2 is an androgen-responsive cell cycle regulator promoting androgen-mediated and castration-resistant growth of prostate cancer. Molecular Endocrinology. 2012;**26**(5):748-761. DOI: 10.1210/me.2011-1242

[34] Ashikari D, Takayama K, Tanaka T, Suzuki Y, Obinata D, Fujimura T, et al. Androgen induces G3BP2 and SUMO-mediated p53 nuclear export in prostate cancer. Oncogene. 2017;**36**(45):6272-6281. DOI: 10.1038/onc.2017.225

[35] Asangani IA, Dommeti VL, Wang X, Malik R, Cieslik M, Yang R, et al. Therapeutic targeting of BET bromodomain proteins in castration-resistant prostate cancer. Nature. 2014;**510**(7504):278-282. DOI: 10.1038/nature13229

[36] Sanchez R, Meslamani J, Zhou MM. The bromodomain: From epigenome reader to druggable target. Biochimica et Biophysica Acta. 2014;**1839**(8):676-685. DOI: 10.1016/j.bbagrm.2014.03.011

[37] Groner AC, Cato L, de Tribolet-Hardy J, Bernasocchi T, Janouskova H, Melchers D, et al. TRIM24 is an oncogenic transcriptional activator in prostate cancer. Cancer Cell. 2016;**29**(6):846-858. DOI: 10.1016/j.ccell.2016

[38] Zhang P, Wang D, Zhao Y, Ren S, Gao K, Ye Z, et al. Intrinsic BET inhibitor resistance in SPOP-mutated prostate cancer is mediated by BET protein stabilization and AKT-mTORC1 activation. Nature Medicine. 2017;**23**(9):1055-1062. DOI: 10.1038/nm.4379

[39] Takayama K, Tsutsumi S, Katayama S, Okayama T, Horie-Inoue K, Ikeda K, et al. Integration of cap analysis of gene expression and chromatin immunoprecipitation analysis on array reveals genome-wide androgen receptor signaling in prostate cancer cells. Oncogene. 2011;**30**(5):619-630. DOI: 10.1038/onc.2010.436

[40] Eissenberg JC, Shilatifard A. Histone H3 lysine 4 (H3K4) methylation in development and differentiation. Developmental Biology. 2010;**339**:240-249. DOI: 10.1016/j.ydbio.2009.08.017

[41] Malik R, Khan AP, Asangani IA, Cieślik M, Prensner JR, Wang X, et al. Targeting the MLL complex in castration-resistant prostate cancer. Nature Medicine. 2015;**21**(4):344-352. DOI: 10.1038/nm.3830

[42] Metzger E, Yin N, Wissmann M, Kunowska N, Fischer K, Friedrichs N, et al. Phosphorylation of histone H3 at threonine 11 establishes a novel chromatin mark for transcriptional regulation. Nature Cell Biology. 2008;**10**:53-60. DOI: 10.1038/ncb1668

[43] Kim JY, Banerjee T, Vinckevicius A, Luo Q, Parker JB, Baker MR, et al. A role for WDR5 in integrating threonine 11 phosphorylation to lysine 4 methylation on histone H3 during androgen signaling and in prostate cancer. Molecular Cell. 2014;**54**(4):613-625. DOI: 10.1016/j.molcel.2014.03.043

[44] Metzger E, Wissmann M, Yin N, Müller JM, Schneider R, Peters AH, et al. LSD1 demethylates repressive histone marks to promote androgen-receptor-dependent transcription. Nature. 2005;**437**(7057):436-439. DOI: 10.1038/nature04020

[45] Metzger E, Imhof A, Patel D, Kahl P, Hoffmeyer K, Friedrichs N, et al. Phosphorylation of histone H3T6 by PKCbeta(I) controls demethylation at histone H3K4. Nature. 2010;**464**(7289):792-796. DOI: 10.1038/nature08839

[46] Takayama K, Suzuki T, Fujimura T, Urano T, Takahashi S, Homma Y, et al. CtBP2 modulates the androgen receptor to promote prostate cancer progression. Cancer Research. 2014;**74**(22):6542-6553. DOI: 10.1158/0008-5472.CAN-14-1030

[47] Cai C, He HH, Chen S, Coleman I, Wang H, Fang Z, et al. Androgen receptor gene expression in prostate cancer is directly suppressed by the androgen receptor through recruitment of lysine-specific demethylase 1. Cancer Cell. 2011;**20**:457-471. DOI: 10.1016/j.ccr.2011.09.001

[48] Yu J, Yu J, Mani RS, Cao Q, Brenner CJ, Cao X, et al. An integrated network of androgen receptor, polycomb, and TMPRSS2-ERG gene fusions in prostate cancer progression. Cancer Cell. 2010;**17**:443-454. DOI: 10.1016/j.ccr.2010.03.018

[49] Urbanucci A, Sahu B, Seppälä J, Larjo A, Latonen LM, Waltering KK, et al. Overexpression of androgen receptor enhances the binding of the receptor to the chromatin in prostate cancer. Oncogene. 2012;**31**:2153-2163. DOI: 10.1038/onc.2011.401

[50] Tan PY, Chang CW, Chng KR, Wansa KD, Sung WK, Cheung E. Integration of regulatory networks by NKX3-1 promotes androgen-dependent prostate cancer survival. Molecular and Cellular Biology. 2012;**32**:399-414. DOI: 10.1128/MCB.05958-11

[51] He B, Lanz RB, Fiskus W, Geng C, Yi P, Hartig SM, et al. GATA2 facilitates steroid receptor coactivator recruitment to the androgen receptor complex. Proceedings of the National Academy of Sciences of the United States of America. 2014;**111**(51):18261-18266. DOI: 10.1073/pnas.1421415111

[52] Takayama K, Suzuki T, Tsutsumi S, Fujimura T, Urano T, Takahashi S, et al. RUNX1, an androgen- and EZH2-regulated gene, has differential roles in AR-dependent and -independent prostate cancer. Oncotarget. 2015;**6**:2263-2276. DOI: 10.18632/oncotarget.2949

[53] Sharma NL, Massie CE, Ramos-Montoya A, Zecchini V, Scott HE, Lamb AD, et al. The androgen receptor induces a distinct transcriptional program in castration-resistant prostate cancer in man. Cancer Cell. 2013;**23**(1):35-47. DOI: 10.1016/j.ccr.2012.11.010

[54] Pomerantz MM, Li F, Takeda DY, Lenci R, Chonkar A, Chabot M, et al. The androgen receptor cistrome is extensively reprogrammed in human prostate tumorigenesis. Nature Genetics. 2015;**47**(11):1346-1351. DOI: 10.1038/ng.3419

[55] Garzon R, Calin GA, Croce CM. MicroRNAs in cancer. Annual Review of Medicine. 2009;**60**:167-179. DOI: 10.1146/annurev.med.59.053006.104707

[56] GENCODE27. Data Statistic Browser [Internet]. 2018. Available from: https://www.gencodegenes.org

[57] Prensner JR, Chinnaiyan AM. The emergence of lncRNAs in cancer biology. Cancer Discovery. 2011;**1**:391-407. DOI: 10.1158/2159-8290.CD-11-0209

[58] Wang D, Garcia-Bassets I, Benner C, Li W, Su X, Zhou Y, et al. Reprogramming transcription by distinct classes of enhancers functionally defined by eRNA. Nature. 2011;**474**:390-394. DOI: 10.1038/nature10006

[59] Hsieh CL, Fei T, Chen Y, Li T, Gao Y, Wang X, et al. Enhancer RNAs participate in androgen receptor-driven looping that selectively enhances gene activation. Proceedings of the National Academy of Sciences of the United States of America. 2014;**111**(20):7319-7324. DOI: 10.1073/pnas.1324151111

[60] Puc J, Kozbial P, Li W, Tan Y, Liu Z, Suter T, et al. Ligand-dependent enhancer activation regulated by topoisomerase-I activity. Cell. 2015;**160**(3):367-380. DOI: 10.1016/j.cell.2014.12.023

[61] Srikantan V, Zou Z, Petrovics G, Xu L, Augustus M, Davis L, et al. PCGEM1, a prostate-specific gene, is overexpressed in prostate cancer. Proceedings of the National Academy of Sciences of the United States of America. 2000;**97**:12216-12221. DOI: 10.1073/pnas.97.22.12216

[62] Petrovics G, Zhang W, Makarem M, Street JP, Connelly R, Sun L, et al. Elevated expression of PCGEM1, a prostate-specific gene with cell growth-promoting function, is associated with high-risk prostate cancer patients. Oncogene. 2004;**23**:605-611. DOI: 10.1038/sj.onc.1207069

[63] Yang L, Lin C, Jin C, Yang JC, Tanasa B, Li W, et al. lncRNA-dependent mechanisms of androgen-receptor regulated gene activation programs. Nature. 2013;**500**:598-602. DOI: 10.1038/nature12451

[64] Lanz RB, McKenna NJ, Onate SA, Albrecht U, Wong J, Tsai SY, et al. A steroid receptor coactivator, SRA, functions as an RNA and is present in an SRC-1 complex. Cell. 1999;**97**(1):17-27

[65] Lanz RB, Razani B, Goldberg AD, O'Malley BW. Distinct RNA motifs are important for coactivation of steroid hormone receptors by steroid receptor RNA activator (SRA). Proceedings of the National Academy of Sciences of the United States of America. 2002;**99**(25):16081-16086. DOI: 10.1073/pnas.192571399

[66] Tsai MC, Manor O, Wan Y, Mosammaparast N, Wang JK, Lan F, et al. Long noncoding RNA as modular scaffold of histone modification complexes. Science. 2010;**329**(5992):689-693. DOI: 10.1126/science.1192002

[67] Gupta RA, Shah N, Wang KC, Kim J, Horlings HM, Wong DJ, et al. Long non-coding RNA HOTAIR reprograms chromatin state to promote cancer metastasis. Nature. 2010;**464**:1071-1076. DOI: 10.1038/nature08975

[68] Zhang A, Zhao JC, Kim J, Fong KW, Yang YA, Chakravarti D, et al. LncRNA HOTAIR enhances the androgen-receptor-mediated transcriptional program and drives castration-resistant prostate cancer. Cell Reports. 2015;**13**(1):209-221. DOI: 10.1016/j.celrep.2015.08.069

[69] Misawa A, Takayama K, Urano T, Inoue S, et al. Androgen-induced lncRNA SOCS2-AS1 promotes cell growth and inhibits apoptosis in prostate cancer cells. The Journal of Biological Chemistry. 2016;**291**(34):17861-17880. DOI: 10.1074/jbc.M116.718536

[70] Katayama S, Tomaru Y, Kasukawa T, Waki K, Nakanishi M, Nakamura M, et al. Antisense transcription in the mammalian transcriptome. Science. 2005;**309**:1564-1566. DOI: 10.1126/science.1112009

[71] Hessels D, Schalken JA. The use of PCA3 in the diagnosis of prostate cancer. Nature Reviews. Urology. 2009;**6**:255-261. DOI: 10.1038/nrurol.2009.40

[72] Bussemakers MJ, van Bokhoven A, Verhaegh GW, Smit FP, Karthaus HF, Schalken JA, et al. DD3: A new prostate-specific gene, highly overexpressed in prostate cancer. Cancer Research. 1999;**59**:5975-5979

[73] Salameh A, Lee AK, Cardó-Vila M, Nunes DN, Efstathiou E, Staquicini FI, et al. PRUNE2 is a human prostate cancer suppressor regulated by the intronic long noncoding RNA PCA3. Proceedings of the National Academy of Sciences of the United States of America. 2015;**112**(27):8403-8408. DOI: 10.1073/pnas.1507882112

[74] Takayama K, Horie-Inoue K, Katayama S, Suzuki T, Tsutsumi S, Ikeda K, et al. Androgen-responsive long noncoding RNA CTBP1-AS promotes prostate cancer. The EMBO Journal. 2013;**32**:1665-1680. DOI: 10.1038/emboj.2013.99

[75] Takayama K, Suzuki T, Fujimura T, Yamada Y, Takahashi S, Homma Y, et al. Dysregulation of spliceosome gene expression in advanced prostate cancer by RNA-binding protein PSF. Proceedings of the National Academy of Sciences of the United States of America. 2017;**114**:10461-10466. DOI: 10.1073/pnas.1706076114

[76] Prensner JR, Iyer MK, Sahu A, Asangani IA, Cao Q, Patel L, et al. The long noncoding RNA SChLAP1 promotes aggressive prostate cancer and antagonizes the SWI/SNF complex. Nature Genetics. 2013;**45**(11):1392-1398. DOI: 10.1038/ng.2771

[77] Fei T, Chen Y, Xiao T, Li W, Cato L, Zhang P, et al. Genome-wide CRISPR screen identifies HNRNPL as a prostate cancer dependency regulating RNA splicing. Proceedings of the National Academy of Sciences of the United States of America. 2017;**114**(26):E5207-E5215. DOI: 10.1073/pnas.1617467114

[78] Mourtada-Maarabouni M, Pickard MR, Hedge VL, Farzaneh F, Williams GT. GAS5, a non-protein-coding RNA, controls apoptosis and is downregulated in breast cancer. Oncogene. 2009;**28**:195-208. DOI: 10.1038/onc.2008.373

[79] Pickard MR, Mourtada-Maarabouni M, Williams GT. Long non-coding RNA GAS5 regulates apoptosis in prostate cancer cell lines. Biochimica et Biophysica Acta. 2013;**1832**:1613-1623. DOI: 10.1016/j.bbadis.2013.05.005

[80] Luo G, Liu D, Huang C, Wang M, Xiao X, Zeng F, et al. LncRNA GAS5 inhibits cellular proliferation by targeting P27Kip1. Molecular Cancer Research. 2017;**15**:789-799. DOI: 10.1158/1541-7786.MCR-16-0331

[81] Hudson WH, Pickard MR, de Vera IM, Kuiper EG, Mourtada-Maarabouni M, Conn GL, et al. Conserved sequence-specific lincRNA-steroid receptor interactions drive transcriptional repression and direct cell fate. Nature Communications. 2014;**5**:5395. DOI: 10.1038/ncomms6395

[82] Takayama K, Misawa A, Inoue S, Significance of microRNAs in androgen signaling and prostate cancer progression, Cancers (Basel), 2017;**9**:pii: E102. DOI: 10.3390/cancers9080102

[83] Ribas J, Ni X, Haffner M, Wentzel EA, Salmasi AH, Chowdhury WH, et al. miR-21: An androgen receptor-regulated microRNA that promotes hormone-dependent and hormone-independent prostate cancer growth. Cancer Research. 2009;**69**:7165-7169. DOI: 10.1158/0008-5472.CAN-09-1448

[84] Coppola V, Musumeci M, Patrizii M, Cannistraci A, Addario A, Maugeri-Saccà M, et al. BTG2 loss and miR-21 upregulation contribute to prostate cell transformation by inducing

luminal markers expression and epithelial-mesenchymal transition. Oncogene. 2013; **32**:1843-1853. DOI: 10.1038/onc.2012.194

[85] Shi XB, Xue L, Yang J, Ma AH, Zhao J, Xu M, et al. An androgen-regulated miRNA suppresses Bak1 expression and induces androgen-independent growth of prostate cancer cells. Proceedings of the National Academy of Sciences of the United States of America. 2007;**104**:19983-19988. DOI: 10.1073/pnas.0706641104

[86] Murata T, Takayama K, Katayama S, Urano T, Horie-Inoue K, Ikeda K, et al. miR-148a is an androgen-responsive microRNA that promotes LNCaP prostate cell growth by repressing its target CAND1 expression. Prostate Cancer and Prostatic Diseases. 2010;**13**: 356-361. DOI: 10.1038/pcan.2010.32

[87] Jalava SE, Urbanucci A, Latonen L, Waltering KK, Sahu B, Jänne OA, et al. Androgen-regulated miR-32 targets BTG2 and is overexpressed in castration-resistant prostate cancer. Oncogene. 2012;**31**:4460-4471. DOI: 10.1038/onc.2011.624

[88] Shen L, Zhang Y. 5-Hydroxymethylcytosine: Generation, fate, and genomic distribution. Current Opinion in Cell Biology. 2013;**25**(3):289-296. DOI: 10.1016/j.ceb.2013.02.017

[89] Takayama K, Misawa A, Suzuki T, Takagi K, Hayashizaki Y, Fujimura T, et al. TET2 repression by androgen hormone regulates global hydroxymethylation status and prostate cancer progression. Nature Communications. 2015;**6**:8219. DOI: 10.1038/ncomms9219

[90] Wang Y, Zhang X, Li H, Yu J, Ren X. The role of miRNA-29 family in cancer. European Journal of Cell Biology. 2013;**92**(3):123-128. DOI: 10.1016/j.ejcb.2012.11.004

[91] Langsch S, Baumgartner U, Haemmig S, Schlup C, Schäfer SC, Berezowska S, et al. miR-29b mediates NF-κB signaling in KRAS-induced non-small cell lung cancers. Cancer Research. 2016;**76**(14):4160-4169. DOI: 10.1158/0008-5472.CAN-15-2580

[92] Nickerson ML, Im KM, Misner KJ, Tan W, Lou H, Gold B, et al. Somatic alterations contributing to metastasis of a castration-resistant prostate cancer. Human Mutation. 2013;**34**(9):1231-1241. DOI: 10.1002/humu.22346

[93] Koboldt DC, Kanchi KL, Gui B, Larson DE, Fulton RS, Isaacs WB, et al. Rare variation in TET2 is associated with clinically relevant prostate carcinoma in African-Americans. Cancer Epidemiology, Biomarkers & Prevention. 2016;**25**(11):1456-1463. DOI: 10.1158/1055-9965.EPI-16-0373

[94] Nickerson ML, Das S, Im KM, Turan S, Berndt SI, Li H, et al. TET2 binds the androgen receptor and loss is associated with prostate cancer. Oncogene. 2017;**36**(15):2172-2183. DOI: 10.1038/onc.2016.376

[95] Narayanan R, Jiang J, Gusev Y, Jones A, Kearbey JD, Miller DD, et al. MicroRNAs are mediators of androgen action in prostate and muscle. PLoS One. 2010;**5**(10):e13637. DOI: 10.1371/journal.pone.0013637

Chapter 4

Effects of Dehydroepiandrosterone (DHEA) Supplementation to Improve Ovarian Response and IVF Outcomes on Women with Poor Ovarian Response

José Fernando de Macedo,
Maristela Rodrigues Oliveira and
Olga Goiana Martins

Additional information is available at the end of the chapter

http://dx.doi.org/10.5772/intechopen.79320

Abstract

There is still no clear consensus on the poor responder (PR) definition, however, the European Society of Human Reproduction and Embryology (ESHRE) suggested, in 2011, the Bologna criteria, which includes, for a poor ovarian response definition, at least two of the following three characteristics: age > 40 years, the number of oocytes previously recovered equal to or less than three, and low ovarian reserve tests score. It is noticed that, despite the use of different effective ovulation stimulation protocols, clinical pregnancy rates remain low in PR. In recent years, however, many authors, including Casson et al., reported the beneficial of DHEA supplementation on ovarian response in this group. Dehydroepiandrosterone (DHEA), a precursor of estradiol (E2) and testosterone (T), originates from the reticularis adrenal zone and from ovarian theca cell. In this chapter, we intend to demonstrate the potential benefits of DHEA supplementation in women with poor response in IVF outcomes.

Keywords: dehydroepiandrosterone, poor ovarian response, in vitro fertilization, clinical pregnancy rate, ovulation stimulation protocol

1. Introduction

Female infertility increases dramatically with age. The delay in the decision of having children is no longer a simple trend, but a reality among women today [1, 2]. At least 20% of women choose to establish their families after the age of 35. This is mainly due to the expectation of the modern woman to wish for, in the foreground, professional and financial stability, waiting for a stable relationship that would give her security [1–4].

Under the physiological aspect, the function of the ovary is to generate mature oocytes and produce steroid hormones that create a conducive environment to fertilization and embryonic implantation, and the aging of the ovaries is demonstrated by reduced oocyte reserve, decreased fertility as well as adverse reproductive events, such as gestational losses and pregnancy with aneuploidy. With age, the remaining eggs age and become less able to be fertilized by sperm [5].

2. Poor responder patients

The clinical management of the poor responders in the in vitro fertilization (IVF) processes is still a challenge for specialists in the field, since there is a lack of standardization in the definition of these patients classified as "poor responders." It is found that in such patients, a small number of follicles are developed during treatment and, as a consequence, a small number of oocytes are recovered through IVF [6–8].

The European Society for Human Reproduction and Embryology (ESHRE) [9] proposed in 2011 the so-called Bologna criteria that establish as a poor ovarian response, that is, a decrease in the quantity of eggs available for fertilization available in the ovaries to stimulation in IVF cycles, with at least two of the following three characteristics:

- Age above 40.
- The number of oocytes previously recovered in previous cycles of IVF less than or equal to three.
- Low ovarian reserve test scores.

According to different studies, 9–24% of patients who have undergone IVF and embryo transfer (IVF-ET) have been poor responders, resulting in low pregnancy rates, or between 2 and 4% [4, 10, 11].

The main causes are numerical and structural chromosomal changes, as well as mutations or variability in specific genes of reproductive aging, pelvic infections, chlamydia trachomatis infections, endometriosis, chemotherapy, and other factors that may lead to the reduction of ovarian reserve [12, 13].

In addition, there is an evident lack of data to identify the best intervention to achieve treatment success in poor responders, due to the heterogeneity of this group of women. Old age is considered the most relevant risk factor, but on the other hand, young women are not free of this condition and may also have a diminished ovarian reserve [3, 4, 14].

Thus, different protocols have been suggested to improve outcomes in those patients, such as: the use of nitric oxide, formed in vivo from L-arginine, which may play a role in follicular maturation and ovulation. Growth hormone is also employed to regulate the effect of FSH, increasing the synthesis of insulin-like growth factor and consequently ovarian function, quality, and embryo implantation [15–17].

In this way, the purpose of this chapter is to describe the effect of dehydroepiandrosterone supplementation (DHEA) as an adjunct in ovarian stimulation procedures.

3. Steroidogenesis

Steroidogenesis occurs through a cascade of events in the adrenal, ovary, and peripheral tissues. The set of reactions is triggered by hormonal stimuli specific for each organ, such as adrenocorticotrophic hormone (ACTH) that acts on the adrenal and luteinizing (LH) in the ovaries [12].

These hormones bind to a specific receptor on the cell membrane of the effector organ, activating an intracellular enzyme, the adenylyl cyclase, responsible for converting adenosine triphosphate (ATP) into cyclic adenosine monophosphate (cAMP). The cAMP, in turn, binds to a cytoplasmic protein (guanine nucleotide binding proteins—G protein), and this newly formed complex is responsible for the activation of the enzymes involved in steroidogenesis [17, 18].

The action of specific enzymes, which are distinct in the steroidogenic organs, is what determines the pathway to be followed. Thus, the combined action of two groups of enzymes on steroidogenesis is: enzymes of the superfamily cytochrome P450 and the hydroxysteroid dehydrogenases. The ovary undergoes the action of the 17α-hydroxylase or 17,20-lyase that guides the estrogen production pathway and in the adrenal, the 21-hydroxylase which is responsible for the production of glucocorticoids and mineralocorticoids [18–21].

3.1 Stages of steroidogenesis from cholesterol

According to Geber, Valle, and Sampaio [20], the raw material of steroidogenesis is cholesterol. Virtually, all cells of steroid-producing organs, with the exception of the placenta, are able to produce cholesterol from acetates in the smooth endoplasmic reticulum. However, this production is insufficient, and most of this precursor hormone is of serum origin. Cholesterol is transported in the bloodstream by low-density lipoproteins (LDL) which bind to specific receptors on the cell membrane of the steroid-opioid organs, allowing cholesterol to enter the cell.

After its entry into the cell, the cholesterol has its side chain broken in C20-C22, by the action of oxidizing desmolase, originating pregnenolone, which in turn, undergoes the action of the enzyme 3β-hydroxysteroid dehydrogenase converting it into progesterone.

Pregnenolone and progesterone then pass two parallel pathways: delta 5 and delta 4, respectively. Immediate reactions are common to both sequences, originating different products.

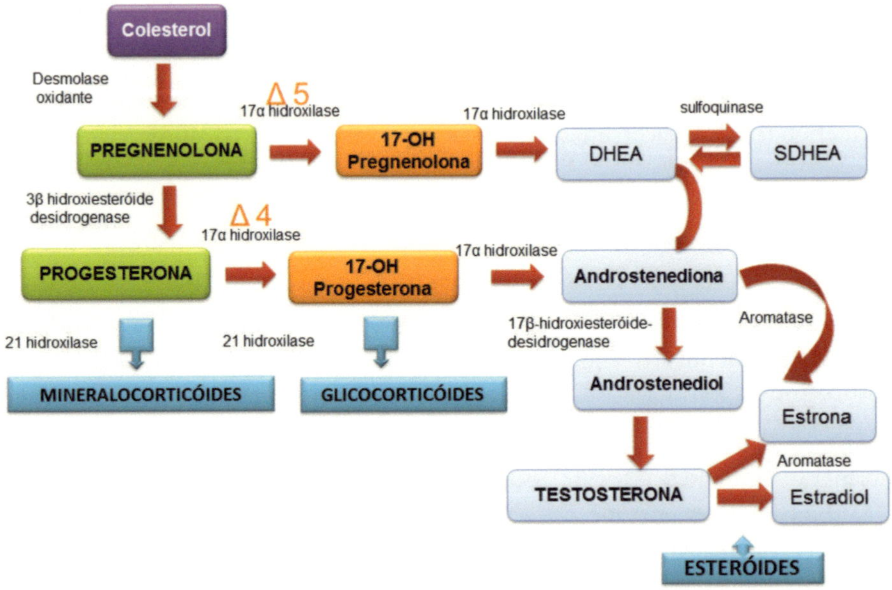

Figure 1. Steroidogenesis biochemical pathways.

Both pregnenolone and progesterone will undergo 17α-hydroxylase or 17,20-lyase action, resulting in 17-hydroxypregnenolone and 17-hydroxyprogesterone, respectively. These substances may be followed by a biochemical pathway that will originate the androgens and estrogens or the one that will give rise to the hormones of the adrenal cortex. 17-hydroxypregnenolone and 17-hydroxyprogesterone under the action of 17α-hydroxylase will give origin to dehydroepiandrosterone (DHEA) and androstenedione, respectively.

Subsequently, DHEA and androstenedione by the stimulation of the enzyme 17β-hydroxysteroid dehydrogenase will transform into androstenediol and testosterone, which are the terminal androgens. Androstenedione and testosterone undergo the action of a set of enzymatic reactions called aromatization and give rise to estrone and estradiol.

Figure 1 briefly describes the biochemical pathways of steroidogenesis [18, 20].

The action of all these hormones is on the general metabolism, thus, they participate in the glucose regulation and ionic balance of sodium and potassium in the body, among others [18].

4. Dehydroepiandrosterone (DHEA)

Dehydroepiandrosterone (DHEA) and its sulfated form (SDHEA) are androgenic hormones mainly produced by the reticular zone of the adrenal glands, from cholesterol. This gland accounts for 90% of DHEA production and 100% of SDHEA production. Other sites of production of this hormone are testicles, ovaries, adipose tissue, brain, and skin [1, 12, 21].

http://dx.doi.org/10.5772/intechopen.79320

In addition to precursors of the sex hormones, they act on the secretion of all other hormones secreted by the adrenal (**Figure 2**).

It is worth mentioning that DHEA is converted peripherally into its sulfate and vice versa. SDHEA is the most abundant C19 steroid, being an excellent marker of cortical adrenal function [12].

According to Rosenthal and Glew [18], DHEA plays an important role in protein metabolism, since it is considered the main anabolic agent, but has an androgenic activity, considered to be weak, representing less than 10% of testosterone potency. On the other hand, the production of weak androgens, such as DHEA and androstenedione, cannot be deprecated because more than about 50% of testosterone levels result from the peripheral transformation of these weak androgens. The daily secretion of the hormone DHEA is about 30 mg in the young man and 20 mg in the young woman, considering both in the resting condition. Food factors such as the consumption of proteins and fats have increased production, while carbohydrates interfere reducing production.

During female reproductive life, the two hormones circulate in the human body in large quantities, with SDHEA having a longer serum half-life than DHEA [18, 20].

DHEA is secreted by the adrenal in a pulsatile way, accompanying the diurnal rhythm similar to that of cortisol, being stimulated by corticotrophin releasing hormone (CRH) and adreno-corticotrophic hormone (ACTH) [22].

Throughout the life of man and woman, adrenal cortisol production increases, and conversely, DHEA, Melatonin, and Growth Hormone (GH) decrease. During the first year of life, the adrenals produce little DHEA. Around 6–7 years of age, there is an increase in levels of this hormone, so that at the age of 20, it is the most abundant hormone in circulating blood [1, 20].

From 30 to 40 years of age, a drop-in level of this hormone begins, and by the age of 70, there is only 25% or less of the amount of the hormone present at age 20. **Table 1** shows the levels of DHEA found in the human body over the years distributed by gender and age group [1, 23].

Due to their higher bioavailability, serum levels of SDHEA are used as a benchmark in clinical exams. Most DHEA, before it is released into circulation, is converted into DHEA sulfate, and that sulfated form can be transformed back into DHEA as the body needs it. In turn, DHEA is rapidly transformed into testosterone and estrogen.

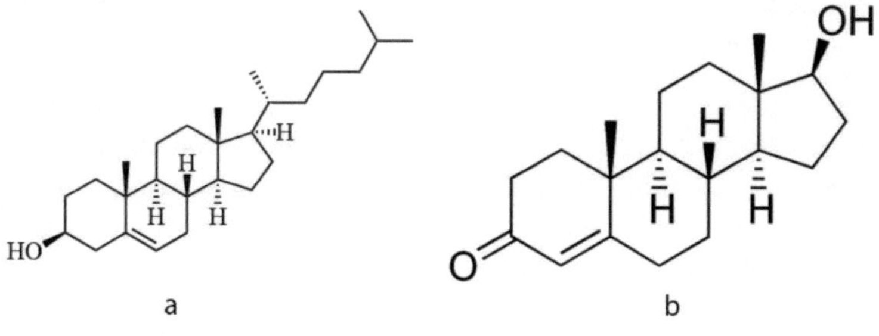

Figure 2. Molecular structure of cholesterol and DHEA, respectively.

Age	Women	Men
18–19	145–395 µg/dL (3.92–10.66 µmol/L)	108–441 µg/dL (2.92–11.91 µmol/L)
20–29	65–380 µg/dL (1.75–10.26 µmol/L)	280–640 µg/dL (7.56–17.28 µmol/L)
30–39	45–270 µg/dL (1.22–7.29 µmol/L)	120–520 µg/dL (3.24–14.04 µmol/L)
40–49	32–240 µg/dL (0.86–6.48 µmol/L)	95–530 µg/dL (2.56–14.31 µmol/L)
50–59	26–200 µg/dL (0.70–5.40 µmol/L)	70–310 µg/dL (1.89–8.37 µmol/L)
60–69	13–130 µg/dL (0.35–3.51 µmol/L)	42–290 µg/dL (1.13–7.83 µmol/L)
69 and older	17–90 µg/dL (0.46–2.43 µmol/L)	28–175 µg/dL (0.76–4.72 µmol/L)

Compiled from: Medical Encyclopedia DHEA-sulfate test.

Table 1. The DHEA-sulfate test measures the amount of DHEA-sulfate in the blood.

The decline of DHEA observed after 30 years leads to a decrease in peripheral production of sex hormones in both sexes. This fact coincides with the appearance of age-related diseases such as obesity, cardiovascular disease, cancer, diabetes mellitus, immune system disorders, rheumatic diseases, viral infections, and depression [1].

Like this, Antonio et al. [1] related that several studies indicate that a replacement of these hormones could have anti-aging effect as well, and some scientific evidence indicates that DHEA also plays other beneficial functions in the body as: increased insulin sensitivity, aiding in the improvement of glucose uptake, mainly by skeletal muscle, liver, and adipose tissue. There is also evidence of the positive effects of DHEA on bone density because low levels of this hormone have been found in patients with osteoporosis.

Researches have shown that DHEA reduces the levels of interleukin-6 and alpha tumor necrosis factor, decreasing proinflammatory cytokines and kappa-beta nuclear factor, which is the central factor of the inflammatory cascade. In relation to stress and exercise, it reduces the production of TNF-alpha, increases glucose tolerance, improves lipid profile, and has a complementary action to exercise, increasing the production of T lymphocytes [24].

Data from the literature report that the concentration of DHEA in Alzheimer's disease is lower when compared to the controls. There have been reports that showed an inverse relationship between DHEA levels and cardiovascular disease and mortality in men as well as breast tumors [1]. Therefore, DHEA is closely related to greater well-being and better physical fitness. In this approach, DHEA has also been used by athletes as a supplement to better muscle performance as a substitute for classic anabolic steroids used for this purpose [24].

Synthetic DHEA is produced from diosgenin, which is found and extracted from wild yam and soya. The dose of DHEA indicated for men is between 50 and 100 mg/day, but there is a danger of aromatization when the dose is close to 100 mg. In women, the dose ranges from 12.5 to 25 mg. Thus, testosterone and estrogen levels need to be monitored regularly in patients who are using DHEA supplements [6, 25].

In women, several side effects have been reported even with the use of physiological doses of DHEA, including acne, hair loss, hirsutism, and alteration of voice tone, the latter two of which may be irreversible processes. In the short term, in addition to its virilizing effects, the use of DHEA may result in the reduction of high density lipoprotein (HDL), interfering with the uptake of cholesterol. Other side effects such as hepatic dysfunction, hypertension, psychotic symptoms, seizures, and palpitations have also been described. In vitro, DHEA inhibits cytochrome p450 3A4 and may therefore increase the serum concentrations of many drugs metabolized by this isoenzyme [26].

5. Therapeutic effects of DHEA supplementation in patients with diminished ovarian response

The possible therapeutic effects of DHEA supplementation in poor responders were first reported in 2000 by Casson et al. [27]. From that date, up to now, about 26% of IVF clinics in different countries have used DHEA supplementation protocols in women with diminished ovarian reserve, and favorable results have been observed most of the time.

In studies with SDHEA, the authors report their performance as a pre-hormone testosterone, responsible for 48% of this hormone in circulating follicular fluid in patients treated with this androgen. That is, SDHEA acts as a prohormone relevant for ovarian follicular sexual steroidogenesis. Experimental investigations with laboratory animals revealed that androgens could potentiate the effect of FSH on folliculogenesis. The authors reported that the use of testosterone or dihydrotestosterone in these animals increased the number of FSH receptors in the plasma membranes of granulosa cells. There was then a stimulus for the initial growth of the follicles, recruiting the primordial follicles early, and consequently developing a greater number of preantral and antral follicles [3, 10, 21].

These findings corroborate the two-cell theory (**Figure 3**), which postulates that androgens play a critical role in the proper regulation of steroidogenesis [10, 21].

DHEA supplementation can rescue atresic follicles, promote preantral follicle growth, and suppress apoptosis, thereby increasing ovarian reserve levels [10, 21].

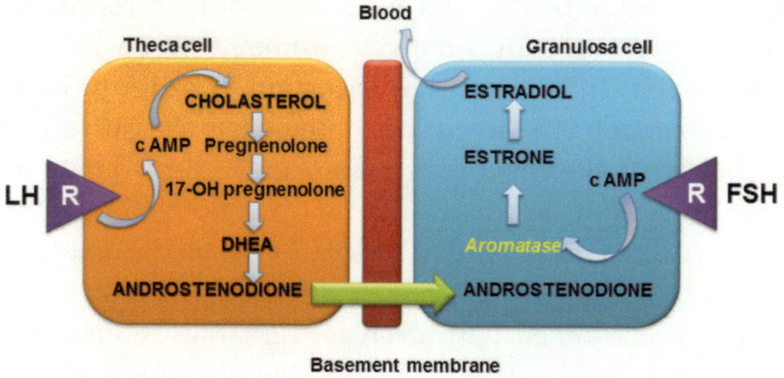

Figure 3. Teak cells have numerous (R) LH receptors and when binding occurs between them, results in the activation of cyclic AMP and androstenedione synthesis from cholesterol. Androstenedione crosses the basement membrane of the teak cells and enters the granulosa cells of the ovary. At this site, under activation of FSH and the enzyme aromatase, androstenedione is converted into estrone and estradiol.

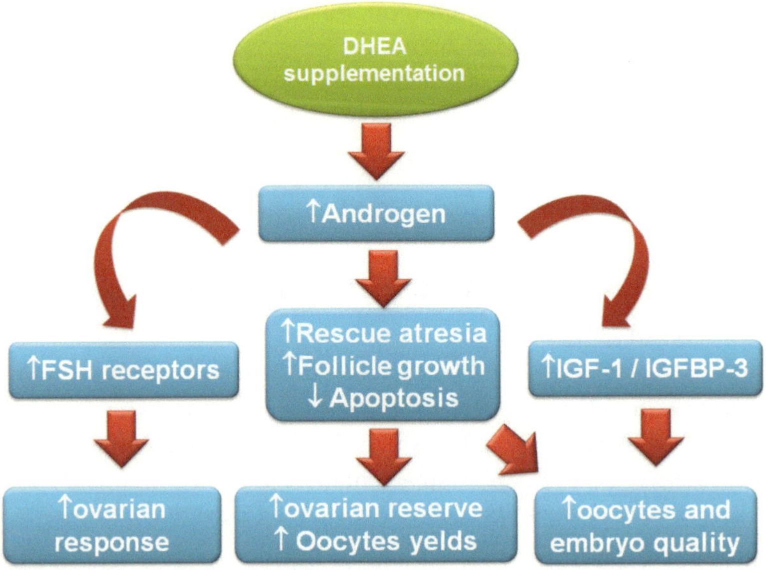

Figure 4. Schematic of the mechanism of possible effects of DHEA in patients with diminished ovarian reserve.

Some researchers reported a transient increase in Insulin-like growth factor 1 (IGF-1) in patients undergoing ovarian stimulation with gonadotropin after 8 weeks of pretreatment with DHEA. The hypothesis was that the effect of DHEA on ovulation induction may have been mediated by increased IGF-1. Thus, IGF-1 is shown to have positive effects on the embryos development, with an improvement in oocytes and embryo quality with DHEA therapy. Administration of this hormone also elevates the levels of the IGF-I binding protein type 3 (IGFBP-3), possibly mediated by increased levels of androgens. Thus, the IGF-I/IGFBP-3 ratio may be indicative of oocyte quality and maturity (**Figure 4**) [1, 4, 7, 8, 28].

Currently, androgens are often being used in assisted human reproduction as an option to improve the ovarian response of women considered to be more responsive. Thus, androgens have been given prior to ovarian induction in order to improve the response to stimulation with exogenous FSH in patients previously classified as having low ovarian reserve. Researches have described that treatments with moderate doses of androgens in patients with low antral follicle counts can increase both the quantity and quality of oocytes and embryos, leading to favorable results in assisted human reproduction treatments. However, it is important to observe that some studies have shown that DHEA supplementation for IVF in women with decreased ovarian reserve did not increase the clinical rate of pregnancy. It is therefore noted that the mechanism of action of this steroid hormone remains obscure and that there are several controversies about it [28–31, 33–35].

The data in **Table 2** show the reported results of using DHEA in more responding women.

http://dx.doi.org/10.5772/intechopen.79320

Author/Year	Sample size	Age	Study objectives	Results
Gibson [32]	16	44.7 ± 2.3	Use of DHEA in endometrial receptivity and embryo implantation	Increased pregnancy rate
Keane [17]	387	39.2 ± 4.1	To search for three groups of patients, who were given GH, DHEA and GH + DHEA as a supplement	The combination of GH and DHEA did not bring significant benefits in the birth rate
Lin [33]	72	39.4 ± 3.5	To evaluate the effect of DHEA administration on the improvement of ovarian intracellular function	It confirmed the beneficial effects of DHEA on mitochondrial function and on the reduction of apoptosis in cumullus cells
Tavares [11]				There was an increase in the number of recruited follicles, of selected oocytes; better embryo quality; lower risk of aneuploidies; higher rate of clinical pregnancy and live births.
Casare [10]	Systematic review		Effect of DHEA on assisted reproduction	DHEA did not contribute to significant differences in the studied parameters
Nearkwichean [4]				DHEA does not improve quantitatively the ovarian response nor the pregnancy rate
Gleicher [8]				Improves ovarian function; increases the pregnancy rate by reducing aneuploidies and the rate of gestational losses
Wiser [6]	17	36.9 ± 4.7	To analyze the peak of estradiol in the day of the HcG; the quality of the embryo; the birth rate after the use of DHEA	Confirmed the beneficial effects of DHEA on ovarian function
Barad [7]	89	41.6 ± 0.4	Clinical pregnancy rate	
Barad [2]	25	40.4 ± 0.8	To analyze the peak of estradiol in the day of the HcG; number and quality of oocytes and embryos; number of transfers using DHEA	

Table 2. Main results of DHEA use in more responding women.

6. Conclusion

The potential benefits of DHEA supplementation in poor responders with diminished ovarian reserve still require further large scale multicenter randomized controlled studies required to clarify such benefits.

The different methodologies and protocols of stimulation and the dose and duration of DHEA supplementation are varied in the evaluated studies. The small population sample and the different clinical interpretations of poor ovarian response may lead to the impairment of the analysis and the accuracy of the results on the use of DHEA.

Author details

José Fernando de Macedo*, Maristela Rodrigues Oliveira and Olga Goiana Martins

*Address all correspondence to: fernandomacedo@reproferty.com.br

Reproferty, São José dos Campos, Brazil

References

[1] Antonio CR, Antonio JR, Graciano CS, Trídico LA. Hormônios no rejuvenescimento: revisão de sua real eficácia. Surgical and Cosmetic Dermatology. 2012;**4**(4):322-330

[2] Barad D, Gleicher N. Effect of dehydroepinadrosterone on oocyte and embryo yields, embryo grade and cell number in IVF. Human Reproduction. 2006;**21**(11):2845-2849

[3] Bartmann AK, Melo AS, Nascimento VCPS, Bertelli TS. Tratamento com andrógenos como possibilidade de melhoria do prognóstico reprodutivo em mulheres com envelhecimento ovariano. Reprodução & Climatério. 2014;**29**(2):44-47

[4] Narkwichean A, Maalouf W, Campbell BK, Jayaprakasan K. Efficacy of dehydroepiandrosterone to improve ovarian response in women with diminished ovarian reserve: A meta-analysis. Reproductive Biology and Endocrinology. 2013;**11**:44

[5] Berne RM, Levy MN, Koeppen BM, Stanton BA. Fisiologia. 6th ed. Rio de Janeiro: Elsevier; 2009. p. 864

[6] Wiser A, Gonen O, Ghetler Y, Shavit T, Berkovitz A, Shulman A. Addition of dehydroepiandrosterone (DHEA) for poor-responder patients before and during IVF treatment improves the pregnancy rate: A randomized prospective study. Human Reproduction. 2010;**25**:2496-2500

[7] Barad DH, Brill H, Gleicher N. Update on the use of dehydroepiandrosterone supplementation among women with diminished ovarian function. Journal of Assisted Reproduction and Genetics. 2007;**24**(12):629-634

[8] Gleicher N, Barad DH. Dehydroepiandrosterone (DHEA) supplementation in diminished ovarian reserve (DOR). Reproductive Biology and Endocrinology. 2011;**9**:67

[9] Ferraretti AP, La Marca A, Fauser BC, Tarlatzis B, Nargund G, Gianaroli L. ESHRE working group on poor ovarian response definition. ESHRE consensus on the definition of 'poor response' to ovarian stimulation for in vitro fertilization: The Bologna criteria. Human Reproduction. 2011;**26**:1616e24

[10] Casarea RCM, Freitas GC, Centab LJ. Androgênios em más respondedoras. Reprodução & Climatério. 2013;**28**(2):80-85

[11] Tavares RR, Correa ILA. Os efeitos do desidroepiandrosterona na resposta ovariana de más respondedoras submetidas à reprodução humana assistida. Femina. 2014;**42**(1):33-38

[12] Pereira EL, Miguel ALR. Produção industrial de hormônios esteroides. Rev da Universidade Vale do Rio Verde. 2017;**15**(2):411-435

[13] Hoffman BL, Schorge JO, Halvorson LM, Bradshaw KD, Cunningham GF. Ginecologia de Williams. 2nd ed. Rio Grande do Sul: Artmed; 2014. p. 350

[14] Tso LO. Bem-vindo o Consenso de Bologna [editorial]. Reprodução & Climatério. 2011; **26**(1):6

[15] Paulus WE, Joechle W, Strehler E, Sterzik K. Plasma L-arginine concentration and follicular maturation. Fertility and Sterility. 2004;**82**(Suppl. 2):S122

[16] Eftekhar M, Aflatoonian A, Mohammadian F, Eftekhar T. Adjuvant growth hormone therapy in antagonist protocol in poor responders undergoing assisted reproductive technology. Archives of Gynecology and Obstetrics. 2013;**287**:1017-1021

[17] Keane KN, Hinchliffe PM, Rowlands PK, Borude G, Srinivasan S, Dhaliwal SS, et al. Dhea supplementation confers no additional benefit to that of growth hormone on pregnancy and live birth rates in IVF patients categorized as poor prognosis. Frontiers in Endocrinology. 2018;**9**(14). Available from: http://www https://doi.org/10.3389/fendo.2018.00014

[18] Rosenthal MD, Glew RH. Medical Biochemistry: Human Metabolism in Health and Disease. New Jersey: Wiley; 2011. pp. 279-289

[19] Stocco C. Aromatase expression in the ovary: Hormonal and molecular regulation. Steroids. 2008;**73**(5):473-487

[20] Geber S, Valle M, Sampaio M. Esteroidogênese. In: Silva Filho AL, Aguiar RALP, Melo VH, editors. Manual de ginecologia e obstetricia SOGIMIG. 5th ed. Minas Gerais: Copimed; 2012. pp. 17-24

[21] Resende LOT, Reis RM, Ferriani RA, Vireque AA, Santana LF, Sá ACJ, et al. Concentração dos hormônios esteroides no fluido folicular de folículos ovarianos maduros e imaturos de pacientes com síndrome dos ovários policísticos submetidas à fertilização in vitro. Revista Brasileira de Ginecologia e Obstetrícia. 2010;**32**(9):447-453

[22] Moraes H, Deslandes A, Maciel-Pinheiro PT, Corrêa H, Laks J. Cortisol, DHEA, and depression in the elderly: The influence of physical capacity. Arquivos de Neuro-Psiquiatria. 2016;**74**(6):456-461

[23] MedlinePlus [Internet]. Medical Encyclopedia DHEA-Sulfate test. Bethesda, MD: National Library of Medicine (US); [cited 2016 mar 2]. Available from: https://medlineplus.gov/ency/article/003717.htm

[24] Santos AM. O Mundo Anabólico: Análise do uso de esteróides anabólicos nos esportes. 3rd ed. Rio de Janeiro: Manole; 2017. pp. 218-223

[25] Dacal JMM, Borges VM. La Dehidroepiandrosterona (DHEA), revisión de su eficacia en el manejo de la disminución de la libido y de otros síntomas del envejecimiento. Actas Urologicas Españolas. 2009;**33**(4):390-401

[26] Yakin K, Urman B. DHEA as a miracle drug in the treatment of poor responders; hype or hope? Human Reproduction. 2011;**26**(8):1941-1944

[27] Casson PR, Lindsay MS, Pisarska MD, Carson SA, Buster JE. Dehydroepiandrosterone supplementation augments ovarian stimulation in poor responders: A case series. Human Reproduction. 2000;**15**(10):2129-2132

[28] Tsui KH, Lin LT, Chang R, Huang BS, Cheng JT, Wang PH. Effects of dehydroepiandrosterone supplementation on women with poor ovarian response: A preliminary report and review. Taiwanese Journal of Obstetrics & Gynecology. 2015;**54**(2):131-136

[29] Xu B, Li Z, Yue J, Jin L, Li Y, Ai J, et al. Effect of dehydroepiandrosterone administration in patients with poor ovarian response according to the Bologna criteria. PLoS One. 2014; **9**(6):e99858

[30] Rutkowski K, Sowa P, Rutkowska-Talipska J, Kuryliszyn-Moskal A, Rutkowski R. Dehydroepiandrosterone (DHEA): Hypes and hopes. Drugs. 2014;**74**(11):1195-1207

[31] Hu Q, Hong L, Nie M, Wang Q, Fang Y, Dai Y, et al. The effect of dehydroepiandrosterone supplementation on ovarian response is associated with androgen receptor in diminished ovarian reserve women. Journal of Ovarian Research. 2017;**10**(1):32

[32] Gibson DA, Simitsidellis I, Kelepouri O, Critchley HOD, Saunders PTK. Dehydroepiandrosterone enhances decidualization in women of advanced reproductive age. Fertility and Sterility. 2018;**17**:371-374

[33] Lin LT, Wang PH, Wen ZH, Li CJ, Chen SN, Tsai EM, et al. The Application of dehydroepiandrosterone on improving mitochondrial function and reducing apoptosis of cumulus cells in poor ovarian responders. International Journal of Medical Sciences. 2017;**14**(6): 585-594

[34] Yang S, Chen X, Zhen X, Wang H, Ma C, Li R, et al. The prognosis of IVF in poor responders depending on the Bologna criteria: A large sample retrospective study from China. BioMed Research International. 2015(ID 296173)

[35] Zhang HH, Xu PY, Wu J, Zou WW, Xu XM, Cao XY, et al. Dehydroepiandrosterone improves follicular fluid bone morphogenetic protein-15 and accumulated embryo score of infertility patients with diminished ovarian reserve undergoing in vitro fertilization: A randomized controlled trial. Journal of Ovarian Research. 2014;**7**:93

Chapter 5

Influence of Testosterone on Body and Testicular Development in Zebu Cattle in the Tropical Climate

Marcelo Chacur, Alex Arikawa, Eunice Oba,
Camila Souza and Luis Roberto Gabriel Filho

Additional information is available at the end of the chapter

http://dx.doi.org/10.5772/intechopen.76706

Abstract

The Brahman cattle is mainly used for breeding and the meat industry. The present chapter had the objective of evaluating the physical and testicular development, and the serum testosterone level of 8–18 months old male Brahman cattle on grazing weight gaining performance tests. In *Bos indicus*, puberty usually occurs between the ages of 16 and 18 months. Variables such age, weight, and scrotal circumference were equally important in the estimation of sexual maturity in male *Bos indicus*. An increase in serum testosterone level occurred between 12 and 14 months of age, followed by testicular and body growth. An elevation in testosterone levels is an indicator that an acceleration in physical and testicular growth is approaching. The variables body weight and scrotal circumference which are important in the estimation of sexual maturity are dependent on testosterone levels in zebu cattle according to literature. It is recommended to calculate body mass index and testicular volume to follow male growth due to the high correlation between these variables.

Keywords: hormone, *Bos indicus*, body measurement, scrotal circumference, testicular volume

1. Introduction

Brahman cattle are known for their extreme tolerance to heat and are widespread in tropical regions. The rapid physical development and acceleration of weight gain during the puberty of male specimens of beef cattle breeds stems from the increase in testosterone [1]. Zebu beef cattle breeds exhibit greater adaptability to tropical climates, as their relative testosterone decrease is smaller than that of European breeds during the summer [2]. The study of puberty in young zebus is of great importance, due to selection of sexually precocious (i.e. below the average herd age) future breeders [3]. In *Bos indicus*, puberty usually occurs between the ages of 16 and 18 months [4, 5], but these males are seldom used for breeding purposes before the age of 2 [6, 7]. Variables such as age, weight, and scrotal circumference were equally important in the estimation of sexual maturity in male *Bos indicus* [8]. The variables body weight and scrotal circumference which are important in the estimation of sexual maturity are dependent on testosterone levels in zebu cattle according to literature.

The American Brahman was the first beef cattle breed developed in the United States. The Brahman is mainly used for breeding and the meat industry. It has been crossbred extensively with *Bos taurus taurus* (European) beef breeds of cattle.

The climatic factors has been studied with a focus on physical characteristics and sperm morphology in cattle in the tropics, describing the decline in semen quality can occur due to thermal discomfort of the animals on high temperatures [9]. The decrease in semen motility, the reduction of concentration and increase the percentage of abnormal spermatozoa are caused by a moderate elevation of scrotal temperature [10]. In Brazil, a higher percentage of abnormal sperm after high temperature and relative humidity observed a higher ejaculate volume in the rainy season [11]. Studying the Nellore cattle concluded that semen characteristics may be affected by environment, by high ambient temperature, air humidity and photoperiod [12]. Studies on the environmental influence on semen quality in bulls have been conducted in farmers with bulls in permanent regime of semen collection [8]. There was a positive correlation between serum testosterone concentration and *potentia coeundi* of bulls, it was also found that animals with higher sperm motility showed, on average, higher concentration of testosterone [13]. Considering the predominance of extensive farming and natural mating in Brazil becomes important to investigate the seasons influence on semen characteristics of bulls raised on tropical climate.

The study of bovine physical development involves serial data collection of body and testes biometrics associated with hormonal concentrations [14]. The male reproductive organs develop rapidly during puberty in cattle [15]. Physical development studies of zebus mainly evaluate body weight and average weight gain [16, 17]. For proper sperm production, transport, maturation and storage, one of the factors that should be considered is the preserved anatomy of the organs of scrotal contents, which is associated with the proper production of testosterone. In [18], reported that the temperature of the testes of cattle should be below body temperature for the production of morphologically viable sperm cells and that elevated ambient temperatures cause a reduced quality of semen from bulls with incompetent testicular thermoregulation.

For the Nellore males, a decrease in testosterone levels in hot summer, possibly due to the freedom of bulls to physical activity, associated with a higher ambient temperature (26.8°C). In winter season, with ambient temperature lower (21.1°C), associated with decreased quality of pasture, testosterone levels were lower similar to [19]. The level of individual adaptation to climate can influence testosterone levels, being studied by this consideration in male bovines [20], reporting different levels of testosterone with 24.04 ± 5.89 ng/dL for the ambient temperature group and 49.85 ± 6.83 ng/dL for the thermal stress group. The results of this study in Brahman raised in Brazil were similar to [21] who performed measurements of testosterone levels in cattle, describing the winter average of 50 ng/dL, in the fall 70 ng/dL, and in the spring and summer of 130 ng/dL.

According to [14], the testicular volume (TV) is one of the important variables when studying reproductive performance of male cattle. In [22] suggested measuring the scrotal circumference in beef cattle from weaning as a way to assist the selection of future breeders. In [14] reported that testes grow rapidly during bovine puberty due to the significant increase in serum testosterone concentration.

The importance of the present chapter on young male Brahman cattle stems from the need to expand knowledge inherent to this breed, as the use for natural breeding in extensive farming system increases, from the transfer to females returning to estrus after hormonal protocol for fixed time with artificial insemination, and from the need to sexual precocity. Many beef cattle breeders still select animals for natural breeding by measuring scrotal circumference and weight gain, without knowledge of variables related to body morphometry, reproductive system, and testosterone level that add helpful information in the choice of these bulls for breeding. In Brazil, the study of body morphometry, the reproductive system, and the serum concentration of testosterone from weaning to the age of 1 year old in the Brahman breed is still underdeveloped.

1.1. Description of the animal model

Male Brahman cattle (n = 40) with a mean age of 259.76 ± 26.15 days and body weight (BW) of 239.71 ± 33.94 kg were evaluated simultaneously during a collective grazing weight gaining performance (WGP) tests, maintained with *Brachiaria brizantha*, mineral mixture and water *ad libitum* (Capacity 0.8–1.0 AU ha^{-1}). The WGP was held on a rural property belonging to the municipality of Uberaba-MG, latitude 19°44′52″S, longitude 47°55′55″W, altitude of 823 m, with high altitude tropical climate, between the months of June and April, for a total of 294 days.

We have previously published part of this work [19]. The present chapter had the objective of studying the morphological and testicular development, and the serum testosterone concentration of 8–18 months old Brahman males on grazing weight gaining performance tests, to assist in the selection of young bulls. The results could be extrapolated from a global context.

2. Correlation of testosterone with body weight and morphometry of the reproductive system

An increase in serum testosterone level occurred between 12 and 14 months of age, followed by testicular and body growth. An elevation in testosterone levels is an indicator that an acceleration in physical and testicular growth is approaching. For body weight (BW), scrotal circumference (SC) and girth (G), there were differences ($P < 0.05$) between the ages of 12, 14, and

16 months, with increasing values (**Table 1** and **Figure 1**). At 10 months of age, all variables exhibited similar behaviors, with increase observed between 12 and 16 months.

The behavior emphasizes the importance of verifying the correlation between these variables, which can be seen in **Table 2**.

Collection	Age (months)	Weight (kg)	SC (cm)	G (m)
1	8	239.71 ± 33.94 C	.....	.....
2	10	261.76 ± 29.76 C	21.31 ± 1.83 C	1.46 ± 0.06 C
3	12	252.38 ± 30.16 C	22.11 ± 2.14 C	1.48 ± 0.06 C
4	14	298.46 ± 27.78 B	23.96 ± 2.55 B	1.55 ± 0.06 B
5	16	353.60 ± 29.66 A	26.76 ± 2.58 A	1.65 ± 0.05 A
6	18	378.16 ± 31.49 A	27.77 ± 2.77 A	1.70 ± 0.08 A

Legend: A, B, C - Capital letters in different columns differ among themselves (P <0.05).

Table 1. Mean values and standard deviations for body weight (W), scrotal circumference (SC) and girth (G) measured every 56 days in male Brahman breed animals aged between 259 days (1st collection) and 497 days (6th collection), created extensively in collective grazing weight gaining performance tests, Uberaba-MG.

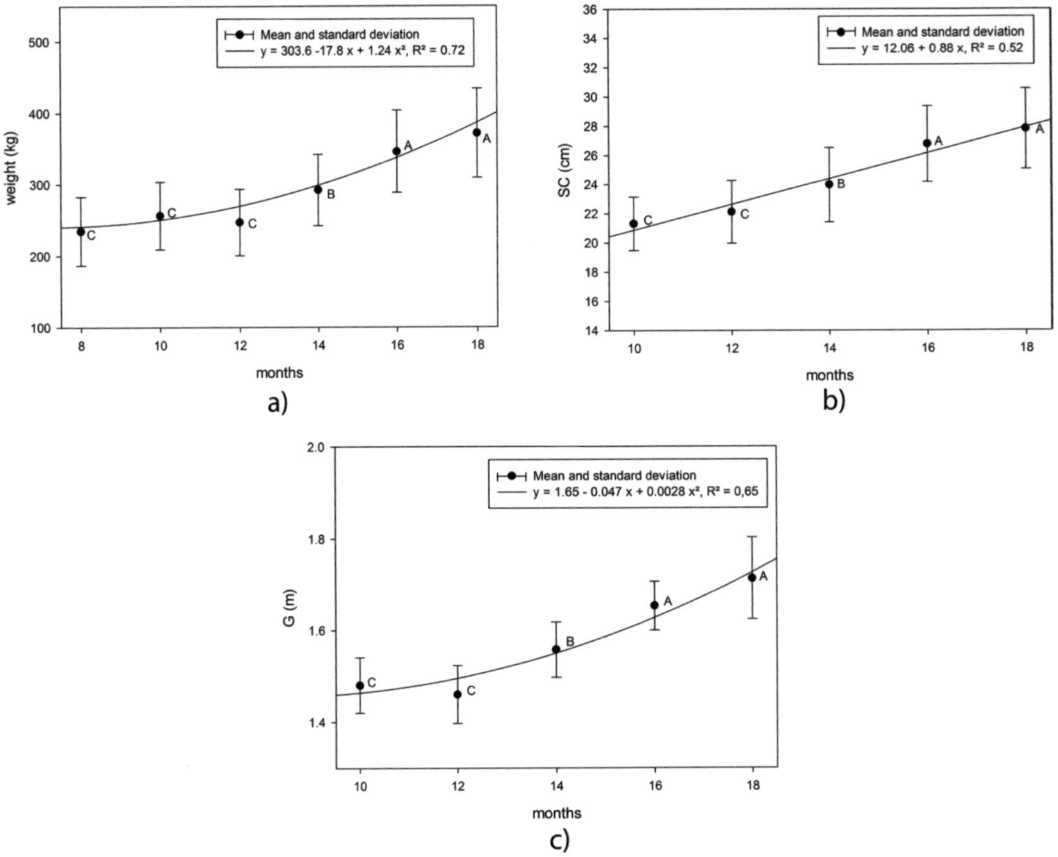

Figure 1. Polynomial models of body weight (W) (quadratic), scrotal circumference (SC) (linear) and girth (G) (quadratic) as a function of animal age. (A) Weight, (B) SC and (C) G.

	SC	G	WH	BL	BMI	ADG	RTL	RTH	LTL	LTH	TV	ST
Weight	0.83	-	-	-	0.76	0.36	0.64	0.81	0.56	0.75	0.71	0.56
SC		-	-	-	0.65	0.50	0.79	0.91	0.75	0.90	0.91	0.41
TP			1	1	-0.46	-	-	-	-	-	-	0.34
WH				1	-0.46	-	-	-	-	-	-	0.39
BL					-0.46	-	-	-	-	-	-	0.40
BMI						0.62	0.43	0.61	0.42	0.62	0.52	0.40
ADG							0.54	0.65	0.45	0.56	0.57	-
RTL								0.74	0.85	0.70	0.89	-
RTH									0.68	0.93	0.87	0.23
LTL										0.72	0.87	-
LTH											0.87	0.21
TV												0.22

Legend: variable pairs with a positive correlation coefficient tend to increase together; variable pairs with negative correlation coefficients, one variable tends to decrease as the other increases. For pairs with the "-" symbol, there is no relationship between the two variables, P <0.05.

Table 2. Significant correlations (P < 0.01) between the physical and testicular biometric characteristics measured every 56 days in male Brahman cattle aged between 259 days (1st collection) and 497 days (6th collection), raised extensively in collective grazing weight gaining performance tests, Uberaba-MG. 2012/2013.

The same table shows correlation between these variables, between scrotal circumference and body weight (0.85). Thus, a curve for the prediction of scrotal circumference as a function of body weight can be generated, creating a prediction model to help producers and researchers determine scrotal circumference as a function of body weight (**Figure 2a**). It is worth mentioning the correlation between the variables body weight and testosterone level (ST), the highest correlation (0.56) found for the latter variable, which similarly justified a testosterone level prediction curve as a function of body weight (**Figure 2b**).

As the Brahman bulls kept growing, several significant positive correlations between body morphometry and reproductive organs variables were expected. According to **Table 2**, there was a high correlation between testicular volume (TV) and body weight (r = 0.70; P < 0.01); TV × scrotal circumference (r = 0.90; P < 0.01), and TV × body mass index (r = 0.93; P < 0.01). Positive correlations (P < 0.01) were also observed between scrotal circumference and age (r = 0.72), body weight (r = 0.83), testicular length (r = 0.74), and testicular height (r = 0.89).

Positive correlations asserted the influence of testosterone on body morphometry: testosterone ST × G (r = 0.38; P < 0.01); testosterone ST × weight WH (r = 0.38; P < 0.01); testosterone ST × right testicle RTH (r = 0.23; P < 0.05); testosterone ST × left testicle LTH (r = 0.21; P < 0.01); and testosterone ST × testicular volume TV (r = 0.22; P < 0.008) (**Table 2**).

For height at the withers (WH), body length (BL), and body mass index (BMI), the behavior is analogous to mean differences with male age, with differences (P < 0.05) between 14 and 16 months (**Table 3** and **Figure 3**). It is worth noting that the only correlation with scrotal circumference is given by the body mass index variable (r = 0.76) (**Table 2**). This result is expected, since body mass index is obtained directly from the body weight, and also by the

Collection	Age (months)	WH (m)	BL (m)	BMI (kg. m^{-2})
1	8	.....	.....	.....
2	10	1.16 ± 0.03 B	1.19 ± 0.04 B	193.15 ± 16.74 B
3	12	1.17 ± 0.03 B	1.21 ± 0.04 B	181.55 ± 16.80 B
4	14	1.18 ± 0.03 B	1.21 ± 0.04 B	212.05 ± 15.60 B
5	16	1.24 ± 0.04 A	1.29 ± 0.03 A	227.90 ± 17.05 A
6	18	1.26 ± 0.03 A	1.29 ± 0.04 A	236.87 ± 18.02 A

Legend: A, B, C - Capital letters in different columns differ among themselves (P <0.05).

Table 3. Mean values and standard deviations for height at the withers (WH), body length (BL), and body mass index (BMI) measured every 56 days in male Brahman cattle aged between 259 days (1st collection) and 497 days (6th collection), raised extensively in collective grazing weight gaining performance tests, Uberaba-MG.

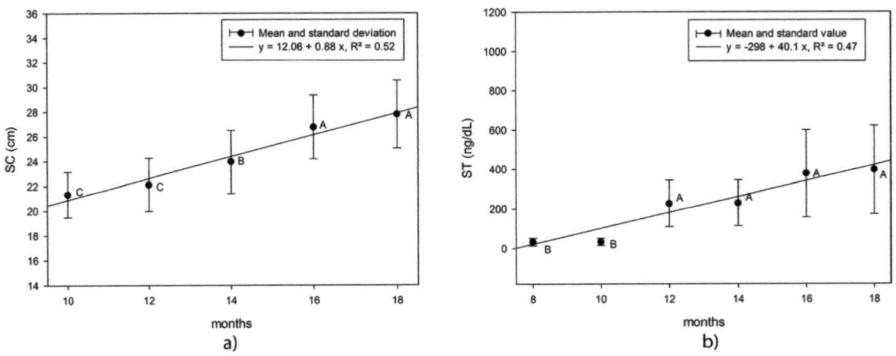

Figure 2. Linear models of scrotal circumference (SC) and testosterone (ST) as a function of weight. (A) SC and (B) ST.

similarity of these variables according to the Dendrogram of **Figure 4**. The correlation of the latter variable with scrotal circumference greater than that between body mass index and scrotal circumference, which does not justify the need to create a model for scrotal circumference prediction at this point.

The analysis of the Dendrogram (**Figure 3**) emphasizes the similarity of the cluster of variables related to the weight (weight, body mass index BMI, ADG), with the group of variables related to the morphology of the reproductive tract (scrotal circumference SC, testicular volume TV, right testicle RTH, left testicle LTH, right testicle length RTL, left testicle length LTL) and the group of variables related to physical morphometry (G, WH, BL); the lack of similarity of testosterone (ST) to any other variable is also noted. Thus, correlations between variables of different groups are of great interest as they reveal relationships that, unlike the correlation between body mass index and weight, are not obvious.

Specifically, it is possible to relate the four groups. Multiple polynomial regression was employed to predict the level of testosterone (ST) using one (1) variable from each group, in search of the one with the highest correlation to ST. According to **Table 2**, such variables and their correlations are weight (0.56), scrotal circumference (0.41), and body length (0.40), thereby generating the polynomial:

http://dx.doi.org/10.5772/intechopen.76706

$$ST = 9236 - 21.8x_1 - 271x_2 - 9545x_3 + 0.01x_1^2 + 0.6x_2^2 + 952x_3^2 + 0.46x_1x_2 + 18.8x_1x_3 + 282x_2x_3 - 0.61x_1x_2x_3 \quad (1)$$

With $R^2 = 0.23$ ($P < 0.001$), and x_1, x_2 and x_3 representing the variables weight, scrotal circumference SC, and body length BL, respectively. **Figure 5** shows the ST behavior upon variation of two (2) independent variables, with the third kept constant. It is thus possible to observe that in males with high scrotal circumference and low weight, or in males with low scrotal circumference and high weight, higher levels of testosterone were observed (**Figure 5a**). One can also observe that higher body length values correlate with higher testosterone levels (**Figure 5b**). The same figure shows that testosterone levels remain mostly unchanged with weight. Finally, it is worth noting that high body length values imply increased levels of testosterone (**Figure 5c**).

With respect to the height of the testes (horizontal axis), there were differences ($P < 0.05$) between 12, 14 and 16 months of age. Testes length (vertical axis) differed ($P < 0.01$) between 12 and 16 months (**Table 4** and **Figure 6**).

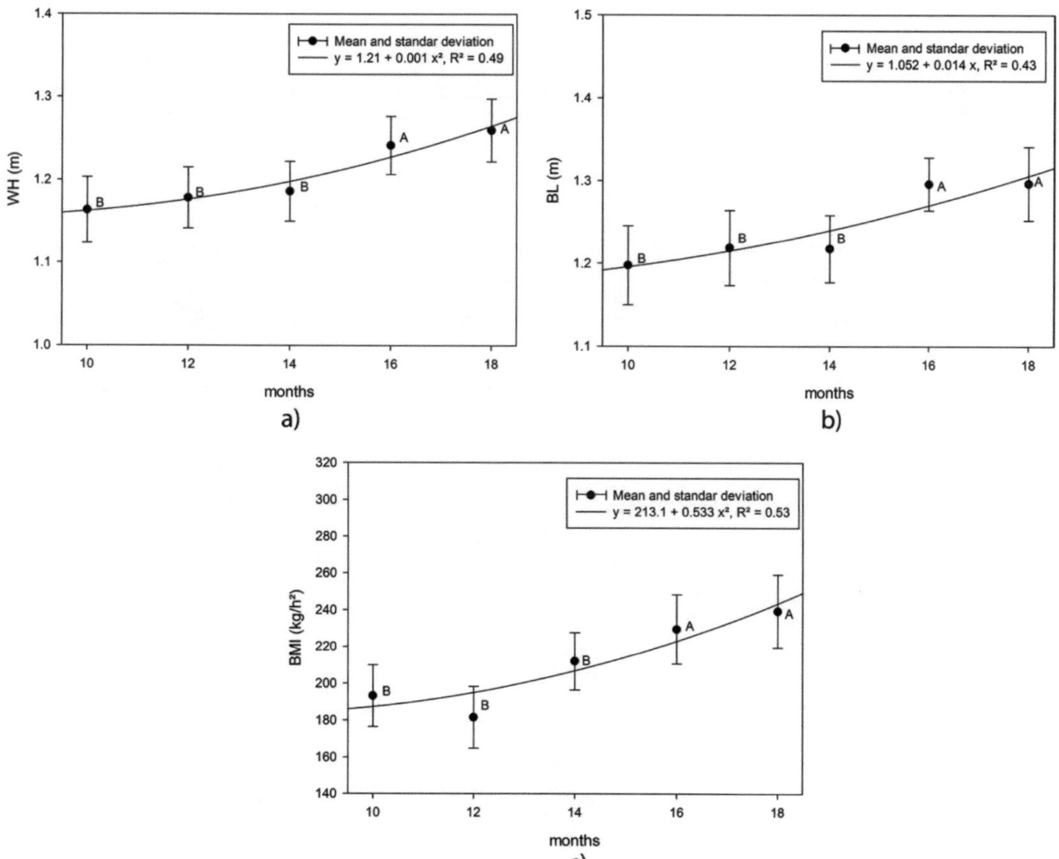

Figure 3. Polynomial (quadratic) models for height at the withers (WH), body length (BL) and body mass index (BMI) as a function n of animal age. (A) WH, (B) BL and (C) BMI.

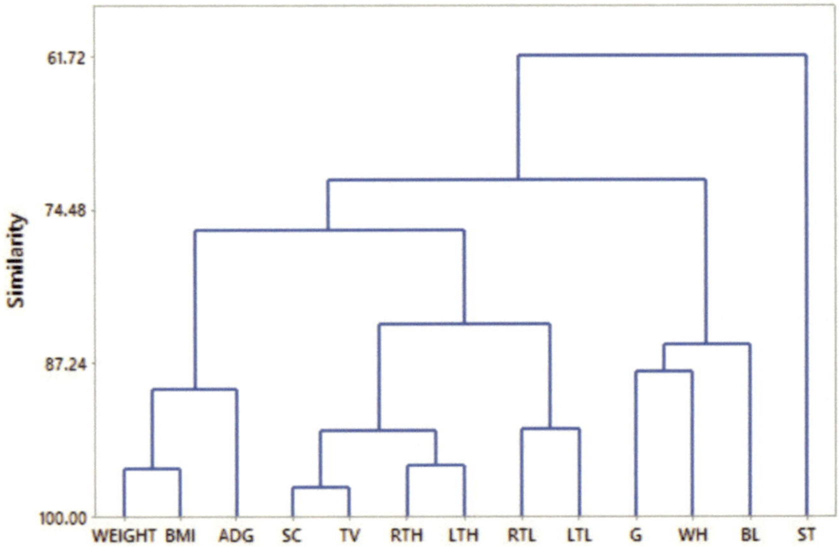

Figure 4. Dendrogram generated by multivariate analysis of variables between the body and testicular biometric characteristics in Brahman cattle males aged from 379 days (third collection) to 497 days (sixth collection).

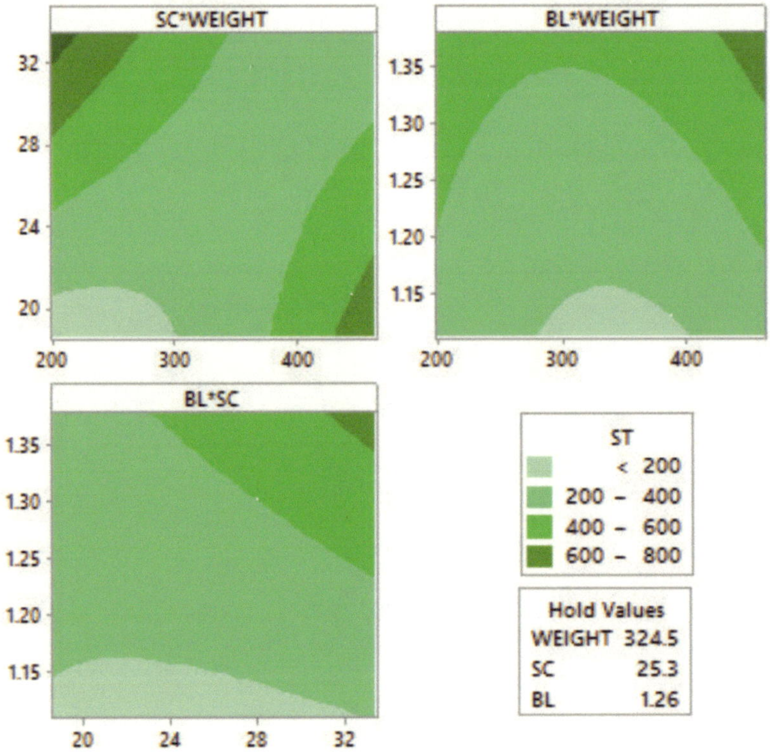

Figure 5. Surface contour maps generated by the multiple polynomial regression function at the clipping planes (a) weight = 324.5, (b) SC = 25.3, and (c) BL = 1.26.

Collection	Age (months).	RTL (cm)	RTH (cm)	LTL (cm)	LTH (cm)
1	8	.....	.....	.....	.....
2	10	.....	.....	.....	.....
3	12	7.79 ± 1.03 B	3.74 ± 0.56 C	7.74 ± 1.06 B	3.90 ± 0.49 C
4	14	8.27 ± 1.44 B	4.60 ± 0.64 B	8.11 ± 1.42 AB	4.57 ± 0.64 B
5	16	9.15 ± 1.37 A	5.11 ± 0.60 A	8.84 ± 1.21 A	5.03 ± 0.59 A
6	18	9.35 ± 1.33 A	5.44 ± 0.68 A	9.09 ± 1.36 A	5.29 ± 0.71 A

Legend: A, B, C - Capital letters in different columns differ among themselves (P <0.05).

Table 4. Mean values and standard deviations for right testicular length (RTL), right testicular height (RTH), left testicular length (LTL) and left testicle height (LTH) measured every 56 days in male Brahman cattle aged between 259 days (1st collection) and 497 days (6th collection), raised extensively in collective grazing weight gaining performance tests, Uberaba-MG.

3. Relation of testosterone with testicular volume

The daily weight gain (ADG) increased between 8, 10, 12 and 14 months of age ($P < 0.05$), but not between 14, 16 and 18 months of age ($P > 0.05$). Testicular volume differed ($P < 0.05$) between 14 and 16 months. The serum testosterone level differed ($P < 0.05$) between 10 and 12 months (**Table 5** and **Figure 7**).

Collection	Age (months)	ADG (g/day)	TV (cm^3)	Testosterone (ng/ dL)
1	8	0.79 ± 0.10 A	.....	32.97 ± 19.31 B
2	10	0.69 ± 0.06 B	.....	33.40 ± 18.27 B
3	12	0.56 ± 0.07 C	154.68 ± 47.59 B	226.80 ± 117.60 A
4	14	0.69 ± 0.05 B	193.80 ± 74.90 B	229.40 ± 116.40 A
5	16	0.73 ± 0.04 AB	263.10 ± 88.60 A	378.80 ± 221.40 A
6	18	0.69 ± 0.07 B	288.80 ± 96.10 A	398.00 ± 224.50 A

Legend: A, B, C - Capital letters in different columns differ among themselves (P <0.05).

Table 5. Averages and standard deviations for average daily gain (ADG), testicular volume (TV) and testosterone (ST) measured every 56 days in male Brahman cattle aged between 259 days (1st collection) and 497 days (6th collection), raised extensively in collective grazing weight gaining performance tests, Uberaba-MG.

4. Considerations and practical application

Studies of body growth in zebu cattle focus mainly on body weight and daily weight gain evaluations [16, 17]. Body morphometry, although subjected to fewer studies, is useful in the assessment of physical growth and development [17]; body development in bulls must be assessed by testicular volume increase [14].

Assuming that the set of physical morphometry measurements opens more possibilities to evaluate body growth in young bulls, the present study measured data from regions of the

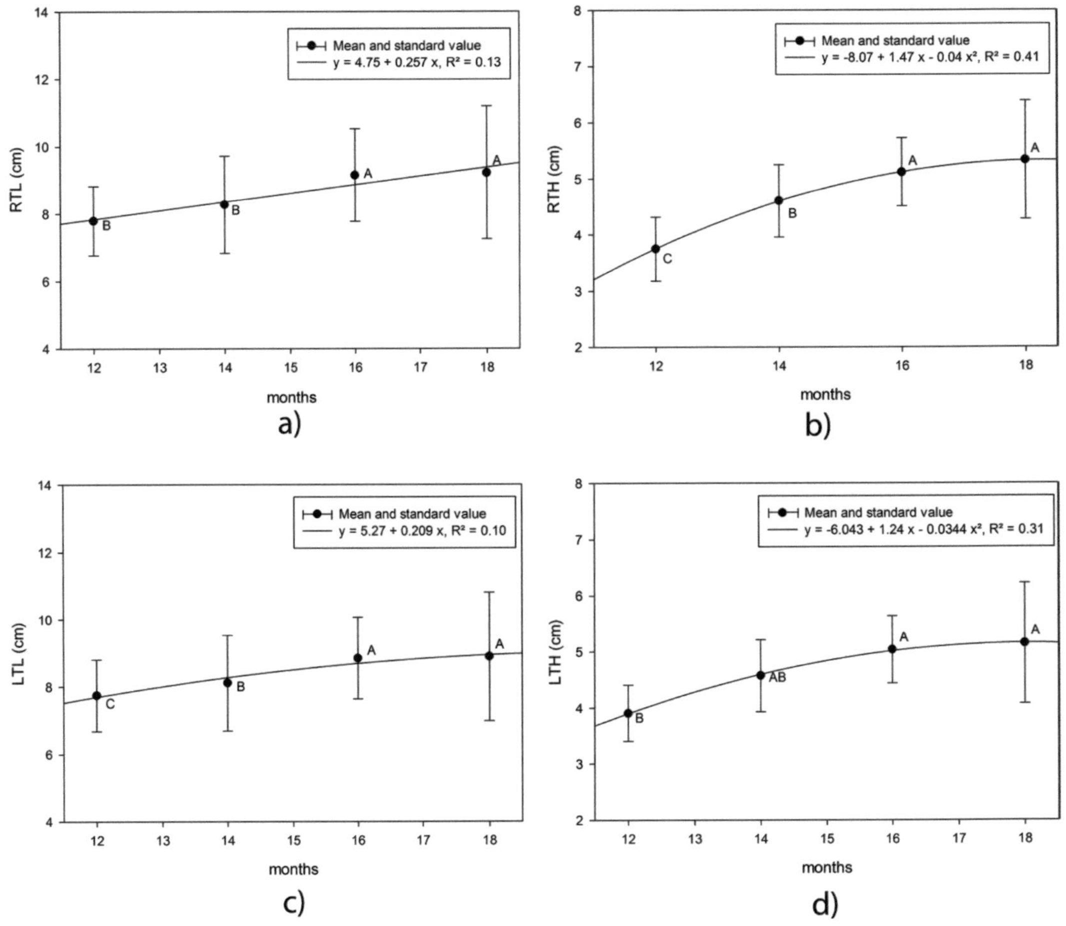

Figure 6. Polynomial models of the right testicular length (RTL) (linear), right testicular height (RTH) (quadratic), left testicle length (LTL) (quadratic) left testicular height (LTH) (quadratic) as a function of animal age. (A) RTL and (B) RTH, (C) LTL and (D) LTH.

body of Brahman bulls. Body weight and girth (G) differed ($P < 0.05$) between 12, 14 and 16 months (**Table 1**) in Brahman bulls; these differences were only observed from 14 months of age onwards in Nellore males [15]. The body weight and girth of Brahman cattle at 12 and 14 months of age (**Table 1**) were higher in Brahman males than in Nellore males [15, 23] and in dual-use Guzerat zebus [17] in the same age groups.

The body weight was lower ($P < 0.05$) at 12 months of age, compared to 10 months of age, probably due to the exclusive feeding on grazing: the quality of grass varies throughout the different seasons, and in the present study the dry season coincided with this age group, in agreement with [23] who evaluated Nellore in grazing weight gaining performance tests. However, there was no difference ($P > 0.05$) between 10 and 12 months of age for the scrotal circumference. Sexual precocity is more related to body weight than to the chronological age of bovines; thus, the analysis of several morphometric characteristics is important to guide

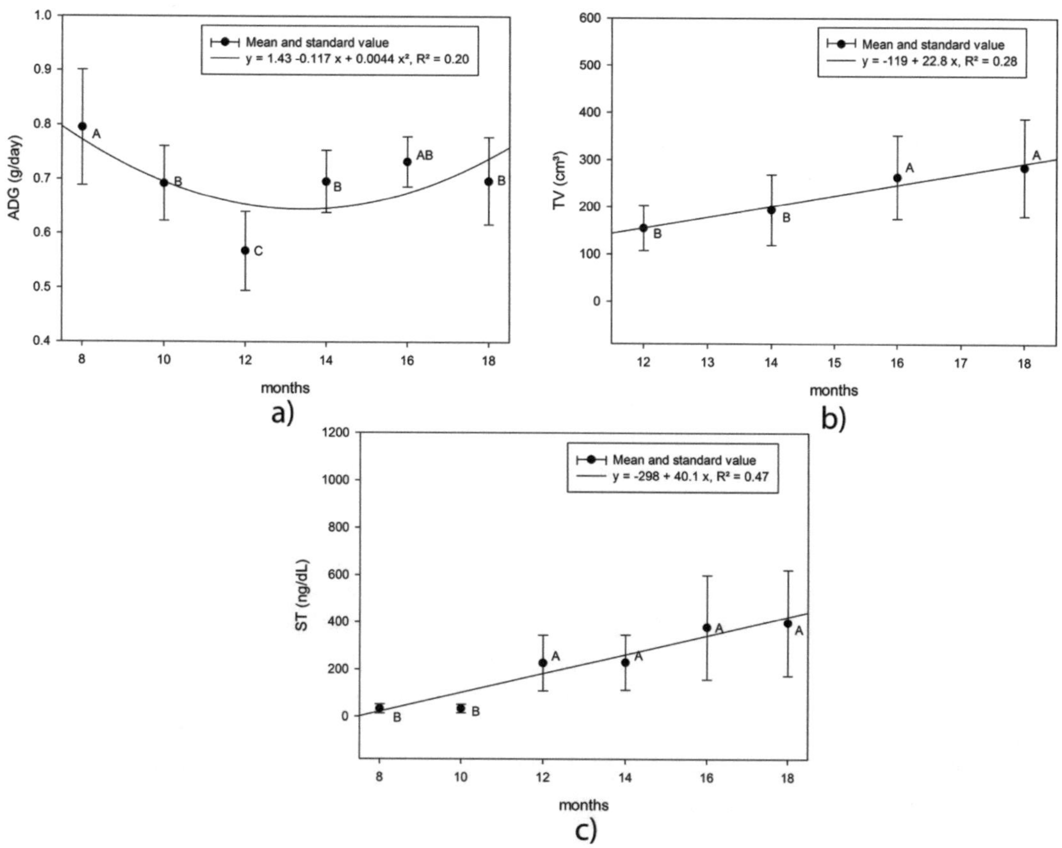

Figure 7. Polynomial models of the average daily gain (ADG), testicular volume (TV) and testosterone (ST) as a function of animal age. (A) ADH, (B) TV and (C) ST.

the selection for genetic improvement purposes [1, 3, 19]. Sexual precocity was described in Nellore cattle aged between 500 and 580 days and between 620 and 740 days of age [8]. The different studies suggest that weight differences at similar ages in young Zebus may be related to the feed composition and distinct genetic lineages.

The scrotal circumference is the body morphometry variable that best estimates the puberty phase in *Bos indicus* males [8]. Mean SC values differed ($P < 0.01$) at 12, 14 and 16 months of age (**Table 1**), similar to the report by [16] in similarly-aged Nellores. However, scrotal circumference values were higher in the present study than in [8, 15, 22]. The significant increase of scrotal circumference from 12 to 16 months in Brahman cattle is similar to that observed in Nellore cattle, probably because both are zebu breeds. On the other hand, the results of the present study revealed that significant scrotal circumference increases occur at a later age than that reported by [24] in Nellore, who reported a significant increase from nine to 12 months of age. Also in Nellore, puberty occurred at a mean age of 526 days with a mean weight of 280 kg and mean scrotal circumference of 22 cm in young bulls classified as sexually precocious [8]. There is a wide variation in scrotal circumference in relation to the age of the Zebu bulls; in the present study, Brahman males with an average weight of 240 kg at 12 months of age reached a mean scrotal circumference value of 22 cm, suggesting satisfactory sexual precocity.

There was a positive correlation between weight and scrotal circumference ($r = 0.83$; $P < 0.01$) (**Table 2**), similar to that reported by [23, 25, 26, 27] in Nellore cattle; in Brahman cattle [28, 29]; and in Guzerat cattle [30].

A correlation ($r = 0.90$; $P < 0.01$) was found for scrotal circumference × testicular volume (**Table 2**), in agreement with [31] for growing cattle, suggesting that scrotal circumference is influenced by race, body condition score, age at puberty, and breeding system; the increase in testicular weight is proportional to the increase of body weight. [32] recommended measuring the scrotal circumference to follow testicular growth in Brahman cattle. Due to the elongated shape of testes in Brahman, the calculation of the testicular volume was efficient: although the males may have slightly lower scrotal circumference, the testicular volume is compensated by the length of the gonad.

The testicular volume variable correlated with body weight ($r = 0.70$; $P < 0.01$), justifying the importance of successive weightings at fixed time intervals in growing male animals. The present study also revealed a high positive correlation ($r = 0.93$; $P < 0.01$) between testicular volume and body mass index, with the calculation of the latter being useful in monitoring animal growth, for identifying average height individuals with increased testicular volume, which can positively influence in the semen concentration. This reasoning derived from the present study, which supports and complements the report by [31] relating body weight and testicular weight; the present study supports the inclusion of the height at the withers variable to track the growth of Brahman males.

With the expansion of *Fuzzy* logic studies aimed at breeding animals [33, 34], one can mathematically model physical morphometric variable studies, attempting to predict how that variable behaves with time. Thus, the present study calculated the body mass index. In Brahman cattle, the body mass index suffered a significant increase between 14 and 16 months. The variable is easy to obtain, as it requires only body weight and measurement of height at the withers as the animal is contained in the cattle crush. By using the body mass index scoring nomenclature for the age of the animals in the present study, adopting the score published for adult zebu cattle with application of the *fuzzy* logic system according to [33, 34], the mean body mass index at ages 10 and 12 months (**Table 3**) fall in the "very low body mass index" category; the age of 14 months is classified as "low body mass index"; and the ages of 16 and 18 months are classified as "high body mass index". Brahman animals in the present study were young, with continuous increase in body mass index due to the increase in height at the withers in conjunction with gains in body weight. Fifteen animals in the present study had a body mass index greater than 242.8 kg m^{-2} at the age of 18 months (**Table 3**). The body mass index was easily accessible, requiring only a scale and a graduated metric tape; it is recommended to calculate the body mass index of young bulls, where 15 animals from a total of 40 showed a body mass index score above average, suggesting a good weight-height ratio. The collection of body mass index data for growing zebu bulls must be expanded, to allow the construction of an ideal physiological variation for each age group.

Body length, like height at the withers and body mass index, showed a significant increase between 14 and 16 months due to the rapid increase of those variables. Testes length and height showed differences ($P < 0.05$) between 12, 14 and 16 months (**Table 4**). These differences were obtained at younger ages than those reported by Freneau et al. [15] in Nellore (15–17 months old).

Zebu physical development studies mainly evaluate body weight and average weight gain [16, 17, 35]. The average daily weight gain of the present study was similar to that described by [35] in Brahman cattle in the same age groups, and higher than the daily weight gain reported in Nellore by [36]. The present study showed differences ($P < 0.05$) between 12, 14 and 16 months of age for body weight, and between 12 and 14 months for daily weight gain. Body weight values were achieved at a younger age than those reported in Nellore by [29], who exhibited a significant increase in body weight between 15 and 16 months of age. Although both the Brahman and Nellore breeds are zebu breeds, the difference may stem from the different geographical locations of the studies.

Testicular volume was described as a suitable variable for the evaluation of post-pubertal *Bos indicus* males [8]. Measurements of the length, width and height of the testes axes are useful for evaluating testicular symmetry and calculating testes volume [23, 37]. At 12 and 18 months of age, the length, width and volume of testes were higher than the values reported in Nellore cattle by [23] at the same age groups. The testicular volume differed ($P < 0.05$) between 14 and 16 months (**Table 5**). This difference was obtained later than in the studies by [26], who described larger testicular development between 10 and 16 months of age, with a significant development between 10 and 11 months, and [29] who observed a greater variation of the SC from 10 months of age. Since the scrotal circumference is used in the calculation of the testicular volume, the former influences testicular volumetry; thus, In [23] suggested that in Zebus, who generally exhibit elongated testes, testicular volume and scrotal circumference should be adopted simultaneously to evaluate growth.

The rapid body development and acceleration of weight gain in the puberty of male beef breed cattle is associated with the increase in testosterone production [1]. Zebu breeds exhibit greater adaptability to the tropical climate, with a lower relative testosterone decrease in the summer compared to European breed bulls [38].

The serum testosterone differed ($P < 0.05$) between 10 and 12 months (**Table 5**), preceding a significant increase in morphological variables. At 12 months of age, the serum testosterone concentration in Brahman males was similar to that found in Nellore cattle aged 31 and 35 months by [37], and in crossbred Holstein × Thaparkar males between 9 and 12 months of age by [3]. In the present study, Brahman males produced similar levels of testosterone at younger ages than Zebus [37], and in the same age group as crossbred cattle [3], revealing sexual precocity.

High correlation ($r = 0.74$) between scrotal circumference and serum testosterone was observed, highlighting the hormonal influence on the development of testes. In agreement with [14, 29], the elevation of testosterone occurs prior to the rapid growth of the testes. Testicular development occurs slowly before the significant increase of the testosterone; gonad growth peaks during puberty, followed once more by slow growth, indicative of sexual maturity. In the present study, the high positive correlation between the concentration of testosterone and scrotal circumference renders measurement of the latter a good indicator of puberty, confirming reports by [1, 2, 8].

In growing Brahman males, the evaluated morphometric variables were useful to follow the physical development. From 12 to 14 months, body weight, scrotal circumference and girth increased rapidly, while the other variables rose significantly at 14 months of age. Due to the growth of the animals, high positive correlations were found between physical and testicular morphometric variables. There was a correlation between age and weight ($r = 0.80$; $P < 0.01$), similar to that described in Brahman cattle [32]. At the ages of 16 and 18 months, scrotal circumference and body weight values were similar to and higher than those reported in Nellore by [38], respectively.

5. Conclusions

In young Brahman bulls an increase in serum testosterone level occurred between 12 and 14 months of age, followed by testicular and body growth. An elevation in testosterone levels is an indicator that an acceleration in physical and testicular growth is approaching. The testicular development and the serum testosterone concentration differ between Brahman and *Bos taurus*. In view of the results presented herein, the present chapter contributes with the Brahman breed with mean values and significant correlations on body and reproductive tract morphometry variables, which are useful in practical use and in the selection of young bulls bred in extensive management feeding on grass and mineral mix. Regarding puberty, it is clear that the increase in serum testosterone occurs to prepare the reproductive tract for rapid anatomical development. The results of this study provide new knowledge and should be considered in the field of bovine reproduction.

Acknowledgements

Foundation for Research Support of São Paulo State (FAPESP), National Council for Scientific and Technological Development and the Brazilian Association of Zebu Breeders.

Author details

Marcelo Chacur[1]*, Alex Arikawa[2], Eunice Oba[3], Camila Souza[2] and Luis Roberto Gabriel Filho[4]

*Address all correspondence to: marcelo.chacur@uol.com.br

1 University of Western São Paulo, UNOESTE, President Prudente, Brazil

2 UNOESTE, President Prudente, Brazil

3 University of São Paulo State, UNESP, Botucatu, Brazil

4 University of São Paulo State, UNESP, Tupã, Brazil

References

[1] Reddy VB, Sivakumar AS, Jeong DW, Woo YB, Park SJ, Lee SY, Byun JW, Kim CH, Cho SY, Hwang I. Beef quality traits of heifer in comparison with steer, bull and cow at various feeding envinronments. Animal Science Journal. 2014;**86**:1-16. DOI: 10.1111/asj.12266

[2] Quezada-casasola A, Martínez-armendáliz KE, Carrera-chávez JM, Pérez-eguía E, Rodríguez-alarcón CA, Avendaño-reyes L. Effect of season on scrotal circumference, semen characteristics and testosterone serum concentration in Mexican Corriente and other beef breed bulls. Animal Reproduction. 2016;**13**:787-794. DOI: 10.21451/1984-3143-AR805

[3] Kumar B, Pandita S, Prakash BS, Mallick S, Mili B. Responsiveness of prepubertal cross-bred bull calves to exogenous GnRH and its impacts on reproductive hormones under on tropical conditions. Springer Plus. 2016;**8**:288-292. DOI: 10.1186/s40064-016-1956-4

[4] Wolf FR, Almquist JO, Hale EB. Prepuberal behaviour and puberal characteristics of beef bulls on high nutrient allowance. Journal of Animal Science. 1965;**24**:761-765 https://doi.org/10.2527/jas1965.243761x

[5] Lunstra DD, Ford JJ, Echternkamp SE. Puberty in beef bulls: Hormone concentrations, growth, testicular development, sperm production and sexual aggressiveness in bulls of different breeds. Journal of Animal Science. 1978;**46**:1054-1062. DOI: 10.5433/1679-0359.2017v38n4Supl1p2561

[6] Chenoweth JP, Chase CC Jr, MJD T, Wilcox CJ, Larsen RE. Breed and other effects on reproductive traits and breeding soundness categorization in young beef bulls in Florida. Theriogenology. 1996;**46**:1159-1170 https://doi.org/10.1016/S0093-691X(96)00287-7

[7] ValefilhoVR,BergmannJAG,AndradeVJ,QuirinoCR,ReisSR,MendonçaRMA.Andrologic characterization of Nelore bulls selected for the first breed season. Revista Brasileira de Reprodução Animal. 1997;**21**:42-44. DOI: 10.5433/1679-0359.2017v38n4Supl1p2561

[8] Brito LFC, Silva AEDF, Unanian MM, Dode MAN, Barbosa RT, Kastelic JP. Sexual development and early- and late-maturing *Bos indicus* and *Bos indicus* × *Bos taurus* crossbred bulls in Brazil. Theriogenology. 2004;**62**:1198-1217 https://doi.org/10.1016/j.theriogenology.2004.01.006

[9] Galina CS, Arthur GH. Review of cattle reproduction in the tropics. Part 6. The male. Animal Breeding Abstract. 1991;**59**:403-412

[10] Kastelic JP, Cook RB, Coulter GH. Insulating the scrotal neck affects semen quality and scrotal/testicular temperatures in the bull. Theriogenology. 1996;**45**:935-942 https://doi.org/10.1016/0093-691X(96)00023-4

[11] Silva AR, Ferraudo AS, Perecin D. Effect of the age of the bull and the sêmen collection periods on physical and morphological semen characteristics of European and zebu breeds. Revista Brasileira de Zootecnia. 2009;**38**:1218-1222 http://dx.doi.org/10.1590/S1516-35982009000700009

[12] Fonseca VO, Franco CS, Bergmann JAG. Reproductive and economic potential of Nellore bulls mating in the proportion bull:cow 1:80. Arquivo Brasileiro de Medicina Veterinária e Zootecnia. 2000;**52**:77-82 http://dx.doi.org/10.1590/S0102-09352000000100017

[13] Anderson M. Relationship between GnRH-induced sperm motility and fertility in Ayrshire bulls. Animal Reproduction Science. 1992;**27**:107-111 https://doi.org/10.1016/0378-4320(92)90050-N

[14] Bergmann JAG. Seleção de zebuínos para precocidade sexual. In: Simpósio de produção de gado de corte; 1999. Belo Horizonte: UFMG; 1999. pp. 51-54

[15] Freneau GE, Vale filho VR, Marques JRAP, Maria WS. Puberdade em touros Nelore criados em pasto no Brasil: características corporais, testiculares e seminais e de índice de capacidade andrológica por pontos. Arquivo Brasileiro de Medicina Veterinária e Zootecnia. 2006;**58**:1107-1115 https://doi.org/10.1590/S0102-09352006000600020

[16] Lôbo RNB, Villela LCV, Lobo AMBO, Passos JRS, Oliveira AA. Parâmetros genéticos de características estimadas da curva de crescimento de ovinos da raça Santa Inês. Revista Brasileira de Zootecnia. 2006;**35**:1012-1019 Suplemento. https://doi.org/10.1590/S1516-35982006000400011

[17] Pacheco A, Quirino C, Pinheiro O, Almeida JVC. Medidas morfométricas de touros jovens e adultos da raça Guzerá. Revista Brasileira de Saúde e Produção Animal. 2008; **9**:426-435. ISSN 1519 9940

[18] Coulter GH, Serenger PL, Bailey DRC. Relationship of scrotal surface temperature measured by infrared thermography to subcutaneous and deep testicular temperature in the ram. Journal of Reproduction and Fertility. 1988;**84**:417-423. DOI: 10.1530/jrf.0.0840417

[19] Chacur MGM, Aurélio PTF, Oba E, Laposy CB, Scalon Júnior O, Inague L, Kronka S.N. Influency of one nutraceutic on semen, testosterone, cortisol, eritrogram and body weight in young bulls Bos taurus indicus. Semina Agrárias. 2010;**31**:439-450. DOI: http://dx.doi.org/10.5433/1679-0359.2010v31n2p439

[20] Chacur MGM, Oba E. Heat stress in buffalo bulls Bubalus bubalis, evaluations of reproduction phisiologycal characteristics. Veterinária Notícias. 2005;**11**:111-112

[21] Jimenez-Severiano H, Quintal-Franco J, Veja-Murillo V. Season of the year influences testosterone secretion in bulls administered luteinizing hormone. Journal of Animal Science. 2003;**81**:1023-1029. DOI: 10.2527/2003.8141023, 10.2527/2003.8141023x

[22] Neves ALA, Delrei AJ, Santos MP. Crescimento testicular de touros da raça Nelore. Livestock Research for Rural Development, Cali. 2011;**23**(4) Available from: http://www.lrrd.org/lrrd23/4/neve23093.htm. [Accessed: 2017-06-05] Acesso em: 05 jun. 2017

[23] Unanian MM, Silva AEDF, McManus C, Cardoso EP. Características biométricas testiculares para avaliação de touros zebuínos da raça Nelore. Revista Brasileira de Zootecnia. 2000;**29**:136-144. DOI: 10.1590/S1516-35982000000100019

[24] Boligon AA, Baldi F, Albuquerque LG. Genetic parameters and relationship between growth traits and scrotal circumference measured at different ages in Nellore cattle. Genetics and Molecular Biology. 2011;**34**:225-230 http://dx.doi.org/10.1590/S1415-47572011005000004

[25] Valentim R, Arruda RP, Barnabe RC, Alencar MM. Biometria testicular de touros Nelore (Bos taurus indicus) e touros cruzados Nelore-europeu (*Bos taurus indicus* × *Bos taurus taurus*) aos 20 e 24 meses de idade. Brazilian Journal of Veterinary Research and Animal Science. 2002;**39**:113-120. DOI: http://dx.doi.org/10.1590/S1413-95962002000300001

[26] Forni S, Albuquerque LG. Avaliação das características biométricas de testículos de bovinos Nelore. In: simpósio da sociedade brasileira de melhoramento animal. Vol. 2004. Pirassununga: Editora da Sociedade Brasileira de Melhoramento Animal; 2004. pp. 1-3

[27] Pastore AA, Toniollo GH, Lôbo RB, Fernandes MB, Vozzi PA, Vila RA, Galerani MAV, Elias EP, Cardilli DJ. Características biométricas, testiculares, seminais e parâmetros genéticos de touros pertencentes ao programa de melhoramento genético da raça Nelore. ARS Veterinária. 2008;**24**:134-141. DOI: http://dx.doi.org/10.15361/2175-0106.2008v24n2p134-141

[28] Mota MF, Souza JC, Machado CHC, Pinto Neto A, Freitas JÁ, Cezaro FR. Evolução Fenotípica de características produtivas e reprodutivas avaliada pela biometria corporal de machos da Raça Brahman. In: Congresso mundial da raça brahman, 2010. Uberaba: ABCZ; 2010. pp. 1-5

[29] Moura AAA, Rodrigues GC, Martins filho R. Desenvolvimento ponderal e testicular, concentrações periféricas de testosterona e características de abate em touros da raça Nelore. Revista Brasileira de Zootecnia. 2002;**31** Suplemento:934-943. DOI: https://doi.org/10.1590/S1516-35982002000400017

[30] Dias J, Andrade V, Emerick L, Martins JÁ, Vale Filho VR, Silva MA. Teste da libido em touros jovens Guzerá e suas associações com características reprodutivas e níveis séricos de testosterona. Archives of Veterinary Science. 2009;**14**:204-213. DOI: http://dx.doi.org/10.5380/avs.v14i4.16202

[31] Menegassi SRO, Barcellos JOJ, Peripolli V, Pereira PRRX, Borges JBS, Lampert VN. Measurement of scrotal circumference in beef bulls in Rio Grande do Sul. Arquivo Brasileiro de Medicina Veterinária e Zootecnia. 2011;**63**:87-93. DOI: http://dx.doi.org/10.1590/S0102-09352011000100014

[32] Vásquez L, Vera O, Arango J. Testicular growth and semen quality in peripuberal Brahman bulls. Livestock Research for Rural Development, Cali. 2003;**15**(10). Available from: http://www.lrrd.org/lrrd15/10/vasqcit.htm) Accessed: 2017-06-05

[33] Gabriel Filho LRA, Cremasco CP, Putti FF, Chacur MGM. Application of fuzzy logic for the evaluation of livestock slaughtering. Engenharia Agrícola. 2011;**31**:813-825. DOI: http://dx.doi.org/10.1590/S0100-69162011000400019

[34] Gabriel Filho LRA, Putti FF, Cremasco CP, Bordin D, Chacur MGM, Gabriel LRA. Software to assess beef cattle body mass through the fuzzy body mass index. Engenharia Agrícola. 2016;**36**:179-193. DOI: http://dx.doi.org/10.1590/1809-4430-Eng.Agric.v36n1p179-193/2016

[35] Olmedo DO, Barcellos JOJ, Canellas LC, Velho MMS, Paniagua P, Horitá I, Tarouco JU. Desempenho e características da carcaça de novilhos terminados em pastejo rotacionado ou em confinamento. Arquivo Brasileiro de Medicina Veterinária e Zootecnia. 2011;**63**:348-355. DOI: https://doi.org/10.1590/S0102-09352011000200012

[36] Ribeiro ELA, Hernandez JÁ, Zanella EL, Mizubuti IY, Silva LDF, Reeves JJ. Desempenho e características de carcaça de bovinos de diferentes grupos genéticos. Revista Brasileira de Zootecnia. 2008;**37**:1669-1673. DOI: https://doi.org/10.1590/S1516-35982008000900020

[37] Ruediger FR, Chacur MGM, Alves FCPE, Oba E, Ramos AA. Digital infrared thermography of the scrotum, semen quality, serum testosterone levels in Nellore bulls (Bos taurus indicus) and their correlation with climatic factors. Semina: Ciências Agrárias. 2016;**37**:221-232. DOI: 10.5433/1679-0359.2016v37n1p221

[38] Lopes JS, Rorato PRN, Weber T, Comin JG, Araújo RO. Fatores de correção para perímetro escrotal ao sobreano para tourinhos mestiços Aberdeen Angus x Nelore. Arquivo Brasileiro de Medicina Veterinária e Zootecnia. 2009;**61**:413-419. DOI: https://doi.org/10.1590/S0102-09352009000200019